The Analyst's Vulnerability

This book closely examines the analyst's early experiences and character traits, demonstrating the impact they have on theory building and technique. Arguing that choice of theory and interventions are unconsciously shaped by clinicians' early experiences, this book argues for greater self-awareness, self-acceptance, and open dialogue as a corrective.

Linking the analyst's early childhood experiences to ongoing vulnerabilities reflected in theory and practice, this book favors an approach that focuses on feedback and confrontation, as well as empathic understanding and acceptance. Essential to this task, and a thesis that runs through the book, are analysts' motivations for doing treatment and the gratifications they naturally seek. Maroda asserts that an enduring blind spot arises from clinicians' ongoing need to deny what they are personally seeking from the analytic process, including the need to rescue and be rescued. She equally seeks to remove the guilt and shame associated with these motivations, encouraging clinicians to embrace both their own humanity and their patients', rather than seeking to transcend them. Providing a new perspective on how analysts work, this book explores the topics of enactment, mirror neurons, and therapeutic action through the lens of the analyst's early experiences and resulting personality structure. Maroda confronts the analyst's tendencies to favor harmony over conflict, passivity over active interventions, and viewing the patient as an infant rather than an adult.

Exploring heretofore unexamined issues of the psychology of the analyst or therapist offers the opportunity to generate new theoretical and technical perspectives. As such, this book will be invaluable to experienced psychodynamic therapists and students and trainees alike, as well as teachers of theory and practice.

Karen J. Maroda, Ph.D., ABBP, is a psychoanalyst in private practice in Milwaukee, Wisconsin, and Assistant Clinical Professor of Psychiatry, Medical College of Wisconsin. She is the author of three previous books and numerous journal articles and book reviews.

Psychoanalysis in a New Key Book Series

Donnel Stern
Series Editor

When music is played in a new key, the melody does not change, but the notes that make up the composition do: change in the context of continuity, continuity that perseveres through change. *Psychoanalysis in a New Key* publishes books that share the aims psychoanalysts have always had, but that approach them differently. The books in the series are not expected to advance any particular theoretical agenda, although to this date most have been written by analysts from the Interpersonal and Relational orientations.

The most important contribution of a psychoanalytic book is the communication of something that nudges the reader's grasp of clinical theory and practice in an unexpected direction. *Psychoanalysis in a New Key* creates a deliberate focus on innovative and unsettling clinical thinking. Because that kind of thinking is encouraged by exploration of the sometimes surprising contributions to psychoanalysis of ideas and findings from other fields, *Psychoanalysis in a New Key* particularly encourages interdisciplinary studies. Books in the series have married psychoanalysis with dissociation, trauma theory, sociology, and criminology. The series is open to the consideration of studies examining the relationship between psychoanalysis and any other field—for instance, biology, literary and art criticism, philosophy, systems theory, anthropology, and political theory.

But innovation also takes place within the boundaries of psychoanalysis, and *Psychoanalysis in a New Key* therefore also presents work that reformulates thought and practice without leaving the precincts of the field. Books in the series focus, for example, on the significance of personal values in psychoanalytic practice, on the complex interrelationship between the analyst's clinical work and personal life, on the consequences for the clinical situation when patient and analyst are from different cultures, and on the need for psychoanalysts to accept the degree to which they knowingly satisfy their own wishes during treatment hours, often to the patient's detriment.

A full list of all titles in this series is available at: https://www.routledge.com/Psychoanalysis-in-a-New-Key-Book-Series/book-series/LEAPNKBS

The Analyst's Vulnerability

Impact on Theory and Practice

Karen J. Maroda

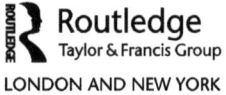

Routledge
Taylor & Francis Group

LONDON AND NEW YORK

First published 2022
by Routledge
2 Park Square, Milton Park, Abingdon, Oxon OX14 4RN

and by Routledge
605 Third Avenue, New York, NY 10158

Routledge is an imprint of the Taylor & Francis Group, an informa business

British Library Cataloguing-in-Publication Data
A catalogue record for this book is available from the British Library

Library of Congress Cataloging-in-Publication Data
Names: Maroda, Karen J., author.
Title: The analyst's vulnerability : impact on theory and practice / Karen J. Maroda.
Description: Milton Park, Abingdon, Oxon ; New York, NY : Routledge, 2021. Includes bibliographical references and index.
Identifiers: LCCN 2021003286 (print) LCCN 2021003287 (ebook) ISBN 9781032040837 (paperback) ISBN 9781032040813 (hardback) ISBN 9781003190462 (ebook)
Subjects: LCSH: Behavior analysts. Therapist and patient.
Classification: LCC RC480 .M359 2021 (print) LCC RC480 (ebook) DDC 616.89/14–dc23
LC record available at https://lccn.loc.gov/2021003286
LC ebook record available at https://lccn.loc.gov/2021003287

ISBN: 978-1-032-04081-3 (hbk)
ISBN: 978-1-032-04083-7 (pbk)
ISBN: 978-1-003-19046-2 (ebk)

Typeset in Times New Roman
by MPS Limited, Dehradun

Contents

Acknowledgments   viii
Permissions   x

Introduction   1

PART I
The analyst as a person   3

1   The analyst's early experiences   5

2   Managing the analyst's needs   33

3   The analyst's narcissistic vulnerability   64

PART II
The analyst as clinician   87

4   Conflict and negative countertransference   89

5   Deconstructing enactment   119

6   Myths about empathy and mirror neurons   141

7   Therapeutic action   171

Conclusion   210
Index   211

Acknowledgments

In this, my fourth book, I find myself pleasantly indebted to many of the same people involved in my first three books. It goes without saying that I am thankful for what I have learned and how I have been transformed by my patients. I am particularly indebted to my many therapist patients, who generated the insights I explore in detail in this volume. It was only after years of treating other therapists that I realized that, in spite of a broad range of early experiences and backgrounds, there was much that we shared. Over time, I developed a deeper appreciation for how this shared experience was at the heart of our greatest strengths and greatest weaknesses. I am therefore grateful to those patients who honored me by relinquishing their fears and defenses to reveal a vulnerability that I believe we all share in some way.

I want to thank David Levi, M.D., Mary Alice Houghton, M.D., Roy Barsness, Ph.D., and Sandra Buechler, Ph.D., for their reading of parts or all of this manuscript and offering helpful critiques. I also want to thank Jeanine Vivona, Ph.D., who I did not know prior to writing this book. Since she knew far more than I did about mirror neuron theory, I contacted her to make sure I had represented her views accurately as well as doing justice to mirror neuron research in general. She graciously read the chapter on mirror neurons, both affirming what I had written and also making some helpful suggestions for clarifications.

Many thanks to my longtime colleague and friend, Donnel Stern, Ph.D., not only for welcoming me into his *Psychoanalysis in a New Key Series* at Routledge but also for his unfailing intellectual curiosity and commitment to scholarship. He is the consummate scholar, embracing intellectual debate and discovery, rather than in-group consensus.

I want to reiterate my deep appreciation for analytic thinkers, past and present, with whom I am constantly conversing in my mind. Great thinkers such as Harold Searles, Stephen Mitchell, and Lewis Aron are gone, but certainly not forgotten. They, and countless others, continue to stimulate my thoughts and feelings, challenging me to formulate my own ideas about theory and practice.

Lastly, I am, as always, grateful for the love and support of my family and friends. It is they who aim to keep me honest about who I am while also inspiring me to be more.

Permissions

Chapter 2: Maroda, Karen J. 'Legitimate Gratification of the Analyst's Needs', *Contemporary Psychoanalysis* 41.3, 2005. Reprinted by permission of the publisher (Taylor & Francis Ltd, http://www.tandfonline.com).

Chapter 5: Maroda, Karen J. 'Deconstructing Enactment' from *Psychoanalytic Psychology.* Copyright © 2020 by American Psychological Association. Reproduced with permission.

and commitment to scholarship. He is the consummate scholar, embracing intellectual debate and discovery, rather than in-group consensus.

I want to reiterate my deep appreciation for analytic thinkers, past and present, with whom I am constantly conversing in my mind. Great thinkers such as Harold Searles, Stephen Mitchell, and Lewis Aron are gone, but certainly not forgotten. They, and countless others, continue to stimulate my thoughts and feelings, challenging me to formulate my own ideas about theory and practice.

Lastly, I am, as always, grateful for the love and support of my family and friends. It is they who aim to keep me honest about who I am while also inspiring me to be more.

Permissions

Introduction

In this book, I examine our early childhood experiences and argue that all therapists share certain circumstances from that period in their lives. Perhaps we share as well in a genetic endowment toward empathic attunement to important others. I specifically discuss both the strengths and weaknesses that result from having been assigned the enormous responsibility for caregiving at an early age. The outcome is an overdetermined precociousness on our part, as well as a deep sense of having missed something important that we needed. We re-live our pasts as we treat our patients, deriving both pleasure and pain as we revisit emotional terrain that can be achingly familiar. In addition, we often favor theoretical approaches and interventions that sometimes fall too easily into either a repetition of our own pasts or a defense against experiencing that repetition.

I have divided this book into two parts in an attempt to address both how our early experiences created the people we are today and how this gets enacted in our choice of theory and technique. Part I is devoted to our motivations, our vulnerabilities, our needs, our sacrifices, and our gratifications. Part II examines how our personal traits and histories become part of the fabric of our theories and interventions. I discuss our avoidance of conflict, our preference for enactment over direct intervention, our misapplied confidence in mirror neuron theory, and how we create our theories of therapeutic action.

Writing this book was challenging, both emotionally and intellectually. I hope the reader will feel equally challenged in the reading of it.

Part I

The analyst as a person

Chapter 1

The analyst's early experiences

Anyone who has chosen to become an analytic clinician is keenly aware that there is something deep and primitive about that decision that eludes understanding. We readily acknowledge the positive and obvious reasons for our choice, like wanting to help others and have meaningful work. Yet, most of us are aware of deeper needs being met by doing therapy. The same is true for our theories and the ways in which we prefer to work with patients. The purpose of this chapter is to orient the reader to the idea that everything about why we became therapists, how we build our theories, and how we practice, is significantly shaped by our own early experiences. I want to begin by looking at some of the early experiences that contribute to our vocational choice. I will then explore the numerous related issues that include our fear of doing harm; our tendency toward passivity rather than action; our ambivalence about technique; our need to see ourselves in an overly-positive light; the personal nature of our theories; and the impact of gender within the transition from classical to relational analysis.

In *A Curious Calling*, Michael Sussman (1992) speaks openly and extensively about both our motivations for doing treatment and the ongoing gratification for the therapist that is essential, albeit largely unconscious. He notes that if you ask therapists why they chose their profession, you will get generic answers about wanting to help people, doing something to change the world, wanting to solve problems, and making money. The point of his work and my own (Maroda, 1991, 2010) is that our true reasons for being therapists are mostly unconscious (although capable of being brought into awareness) and have historically been ignored as a subject for scrutiny—even in personal analysis. Some of the finest minds in psychoanalysis have addressed this subject, but somehow it has never gained traction.

Jacobs (1993) acknowledges that our reasons for becoming therapists have much to do with our early childhood experiences, particularly being the sensitive, empathic child who provides comfort to a depressed mother (Olinick, 1980, Sussman, 1992). Searles (1979) reflects on the common therapist experience of guilt, questioning its origins.

> Thus, it may not be so much that our doing of analysis tends to promote guilt in us, but rather that we originally entered this profession in an unconscious effort to assuage our guilt, and that the practice of analysis fails to relieve our underlying guilt. For example, we may have chosen this profession on the basis of unconscious guilt over having failed to cure our parents. (p. 28)

More important for our ongoing work as clinicians is that we, just like our patients, carry these early experiences and motivations with us for a lifetime. The goal for us, and for them, is not to rewrite history but rather bring it into awareness in the interests of greater conscious control and less internal conflict. As we treat other people, we are necessarily working through our own issues and attempting to overcome our guilt and become the best people we can be. As Kite (2016) insightfully observes,

> I will go on to suggest that the personal history of the analyst, known or not, understood or not, has everything to do with how we live our version of analysis, and a great deal to do with how our patients experience us. I will also suggest that we may become analysts in the first place in order to clarify who we are ethically to ourselves. (p. 1160)

In this way, we attempt to redeem and save ourselves. In some sense, this is our greatest strength—our need to help others. We were rewarded early in our lives for being unusually sensitive and empathic; over time, we naturally extended this skill set into a career choice. But this embedded need to relieve others of their pain can also be our greatest weakness, in that we are prone to taking too much responsibility for their distress. Doing so produces excessive guilt in response to our patients not doing well, particularly if they are blaming us for their suffering—as they often will. Making things more complicated is our potential guilt for what Brenner (1985) referred to as our "wish to see another suffer" (p. 158).

We become analysts to prove, in part, that we are not destructive—that the pain in our families was not our fault. We survive and assuage our guilt in doing so by spending our days attempting to emotionally connect with others. As Celenza (2010) says, "The skill of using ourselves to help others find themselves coincides with our own pressing need to heal ourselves and to do so by finding ourselves in the other" (p. 60).

A supervisee of mine, who had the benefit of being well into middle age, surprised me at the onset of our work together by simply stating that her new patient's history of being unloved and rejected by her mother resonated deeply with her own similar experience. She added that feeling her patient's pain took her to an even deeper experience of her own pain, even though she had explored this thoroughly in her personal analysis. She said this in a matter-of-fact way with no guilt or shame—something I have rarely seen. We agreed that we never lose the ability to revisit our own painful experiences, and she felt hopeful about helping this very difficult patient achieve some of what she had achieved in life. She wanted more for her. She readily admitted to feeling guilty that she had a husband and children, plus an analysis early in her life, unlike her occasionally homeless patient. She also had no illusions of being able to save her, focusing instead on simply helping her to improve the quality of her inner and outer existence.

Her frank admission and acceptance of the gratification she experienced in working with this patient, combined with an equally deep understanding of the potential for this identification to go awry, made for a potentially compelling experience for me as well. Working with therapists who understand their own countertransference repetitions, and who are eager to explore them in their work, makes for both a better therapeutic outcome and a better supervisory experience.

A personal story

In the interests of transparency, I will disclose some of my own motivations for becoming an analyst. My mother came to the United

States from Australia, having married my father there during World War II. To put it mildly, she never adjusted to being here. My father's parents came over from Hungary and spoke little English. His sisters did not care for my mother and resented her for coming from a significantly higher socioeconomic class. They thought her "haughty" with her highbrow British-sounding accent. When people called the house, they thought we had a maid. My mother became wearily accustomed to jokes about kangaroos and questions about whether or not her family was descended from criminals (they weren't).

My mother was naturally quite playful and charming. She loved music and laughed easily. She was warm and nurturing. I loved her deeply. But she was also incredibly sad and lonely. My father was a workaholic, and she depended on her three children for company. My older sister resented her neediness; my twin brother felt overwhelmed by it. I anguished over her pain and worked daily to take it away. When she was terribly upset with us for misbehaving, she would emptily threaten to go back to Australia, then apologize later for speaking out of frustration and anger. Looking back, I think I took on the job of making sure she didn't ever really want to leave.

My story is not just about fear of loss and excessive responsibility for my mother's feelings; it is also implicitly a story of ambivalence. As much as I loved my mother, I also hated her passivity, her seeming unwillingness to make a genuine effort to assimilate and build a life for herself, and her expectations that I would be a consistent soothing presence. As I write this, I am aware of my own warnings about the possible idiosyncratic nature of theory-building. Nonetheless, I think it reasonable to suggest that to the extent that therapists were their mother's keepers, they also would share this ambivalence. (I will leave it to the reader to decide.) During my childhood, I was not aware of these feelings, of course. But I did become aware of them in adolescence, especially in the face of my older sister's rage at my mother.

This is only a keyhole into my childhood experiences, and I have observed myself confronting many aspects of my relationships in my family, including with my siblings, in the course of doing treatment. I will also add that my early interest in countertransference came both from my own intense feelings toward my patients (and desire to rescue them) and also from experiencing my analyst's intense countertransference to me.

The Power of Countertransference (Maroda, 1991) is, in part, my account of that struggle.

I want to insert the caveat that I do not think it necessary for analysts to describe details of their early childhood experiences when they present or publish, since no one is entitled to this very personal information. And many would question this practice, given that patients would potentially have access to this material. I think we could do justice to our early contributions simply by weaving this idea into the narrative of what we believe and how we practice. When describing a particular encounter with a patient, we might simply make reference to some general aspect of our own personalities or early life that contributed to what was going on, be it positive or negative. Accepting that our own motivations and needs play a major role in our professional identity and daily clinical work has the potential for changing the narrative in a profound way.

The fear of doing harm

From Freud's early admonitions to act like a surgeon to current controversies regarding any systematic use of self-disclosure, the theme that consistently arises is that of potential harm. From my perspective, this fear of doing harm exceeds the expectable caution born out of legitimate professional concern for doing right by the patient.

Since most analysts are very decent, hard-working, dedicated professionals, why would such a fear be so pervasive? I think Searles' argument about our shared guilt goes a long way in understanding these edicts. Even if it is suppressed, at some level, we all know that we are getting some personal needs met in our relationships with our patients. Is the hidden knowledge of this personal benefit producing so much guilt and shame that we need to overemphasize our role as not only "good enough" caregivers but also as self-sacrificing humanitarians (Orange, 2016)? Moreover, to what extent is this fear of harming patients a reaction formation in response to the repressed anger that arises from our internal mandate to put others first? Although it is quite evident from reading the literature that our fear of doing harm is substantial, there is little discussion of why this is so.

On this topic, Prodgers (1991) cites Storr (1979), saying,

> Storr (1979) makes similar points about the personality of the therapist. Anecdotal evidence points to a high incidence of depressed mothers amongst trainee psychotherapists who acquired a sensitivity through judging her moods. They also learn to put their own feeling secondary to hers—another prerequisite for the therapist. Making demands often then leads to guilt and fears of damaging others in relationships. Putting others first is the safe option but inevitably means repression of aggression. (pp. 146–147)

Thus, our unfailing preoccupation with being good can be seen as a reaction formation—an irrational defense against our own guilt and anger about having precociously surrendered our own well-being (Miller, 1997). Focusing on the needs of others, and developing a finely tuned ability to instantly read another's moods, necessarily produces a degree of resentment. What child wants to be his/her mother's or family's keeper? Yet expressing this resentment runs counter to the role of soother and peacemaker, and therein lies the problem. I think that therapists of all persuasions have an aversion to expressing anger toward their patients or even feeling it, because it stimulates this irrational fear of not only failing to soothe but also to harm. This is the conundrum that we need to break free from.

Accepting our inevitable ambivalence toward both the work itself (Kravis, 2013), and often toward our patients as individuals, could provide the necessary momentum to advance both our theoretical formulations and our clinical interventions. Even more important is the acceptance that *we are not without memory or desire.* As poetic and appealing as Bion's famous line is, I think it is not a realistic approach to doing treatment. I appreciate that his prescription was meant to encourage receptivity rather than deny our personal biases and needs. Nonetheless, his words are often taken more literally, denying the considerable realities that prevent such a state from truly existing.

Even as an aspirational concept, it does more harm than good, in that it sends the analyst's thinking in the wrong direction. Rather than seeking to have no needs or desires, we would benefit from expecting to have them and working to bring those needs into awareness. One might argue that Bion's words are meant to coun-terbalance the realities of the states of mind and biases that we naturally bring to each session. Just as with all countertransference, there will be needs of ours that arise with most patients and those that arise less frequently and more specifically with certain people. In any event, we all bring our own personal desires, needs, and wishes for the patient into each new treatment relationship, and we may begin a session with needs or desires that have little to do with the patient sitting before us. And even with our work ego in place, striving to minimize the impact on our patients, success is highly dependent on our own self-awareness.

Striving to transcend primitive feelings of resentment, fear, despair, hopelessness, and rage only results in the need to deny these feelings or try to inhibit them when they occur. We are much more comfortable, of course, with deep experiences of joy, exhilaration, pathos, and love. Furthermore, this volume pursues the concept that unconditional ac-ceptance of the patient's negative feelings and behaviors, though easier than accepting our own, represents an unrealistic wish to both have and to be the idealized, loving mother. As Searles (1966) said,

> I surmise that wholehearted acceptance of the patient is another unrealizable goal. We could unambivalently love and approve of and accept our patient only if he were somehow able to personify our own ego ideal—and in that impossible eventuality, we would of course feel murderously envious of him anyway. (p. 35)

Miller (1997) has elegantly detailed our need to avoid the pain of our own childhood through this largely unconscious pursuit of the good parent: "Only after painfully experiencing and accepting our own truth can we be free from the hope that we might still find an un-demanding, empathic 'parent'—perhaps in a patient—who will be at our disposal" (p. 21). This important topic of the necessary and avoidable gratifications of the analyst will be addressed in Chapter 2.

The analyst's passivity

When therapists approach me to speak about individual cases, I almost always see indications of their reluctance to be assertive. Some allow self-destructive behaviors to go unchallenged or allow too much verbal abuse from patients; some collude to create long periods of silence and many fail to press for overdue payment of fees. When questioned, the inevitable response focuses on the perceived fragility of the patient and the fear of hurting the patient's feelings, inciting a suicidal episode, or alienating the patient and losing him. Consultation often elicits little more than a series of "yes-buts" that end with the therapist deciding to continue his or her existing pattern of long-suffering inaction. According to Luchner et al. (2008),

> The therapist may also feel that his or her ability to be selfless is proof that he or she is capable and that without his or her ability to make specific concessions for clients he or she would be negligent and deficient in his or her role as a psychotherapist. (p. 11)

Our rather pronounced predilection for finding gratification in martyrdom can then be used by the therapist to rationalize self-indulgences like extending sessions, keeping patients too long, conducting multiple times per week telephone sessions for years after the patient has moved permanently out of state, and so on. Is there any hope for changing the analyst's perfectly selfless persona? I think there is.

Therapists struggle throughout their careers with a sense of guilt and shame over having their needs met by their patients. Much of the behavior unconsciously designed to compensate for this gratification (e.g., being overly solicitous and parental) is unhelpful. And theory born of denying the analyst's gratification often focuses on transcending human nature rather than embracing it. For example, the aforementioned emphasis on our humanitarian and long-suffering qualities (Orange, 2016) avoids any discussion of primitive rage, envy, or competitiveness.

Alternately, the current emphasis on enactment prefers to see the analyst as a participant in an unconscious-to-unconscious ongoing interaction that is simply beyond any attempt at conscious control or direction. The end result is an analytic persona that revolves around unconditional acceptance and empathy, accompanied by a certain passivity in the face of the ongoing complex psychodynamics that characterize the therapeutic relationship. Much remains to be explored in the analytic dyad, as well as the reverberations occurring outside of it (Wachtel, 2007). I have discussed how the analyst's guilt over residual feelings of responsibility for their caregiver's pain generates guilt-based behaviors with their patients. But what about the degree of passivity that has always been characteristic of analysts, regardless of theoretical orientation? If we feel so guilty and responsible, why aren't we more motivated to be active and innovative?

I think the answer lies, once again, in our early experience. As children, we did not have any real power over our parents. Once identified as empathic and sensitive, then enrolled as the family's therapist, we essentially felt enormous responsibility with little or no power over events or the behaviors of others. All we could do was respond to the situations we were presented with, then make our best attempts to be soothing, empathic, or even entertaining. But we could not change the scenarios that were unfolding before our eyes. One could argue that any attempt to point out a suffering parent's maladaptive behavior would no doubt have resulted in rejection or further distress—something a child could not possibly endure.

A recent, very moving International Association for Relational Psychoanalysis and Psychotherapy (IARPP) online colloquium (2019) focused on a paper on parental loss by Mary-Joan Gerson (2018), which prompted a flood of responses focused on the deep pain that these analysts suffered in childhood. Both their suffering and their intense ambivalence toward parents, living and dead, were palpably evident. And, somewhat to my surprise, the participants were universally relieved through the act of revealing their ambivalent attachments to their parents and by the knowledge they were not alone. It is my hope that this book might contribute in a similar fashion to stimulating dialogue about our early conflicts—creating an empathic environment conducive to disclosing them.

I had a therapist-patient ask me recently why I am so comfortable with giving feedback and engaging in conflict, when necessary. My answer is that my mother, though very needy and dependent, paradoxically also wanted her children to be free to express their own opinions and have the courage of their convictions—not to be confused with them taking precedence over hers. Nonetheless, my siblings and I were encouraged to speak our minds and be aware of our feelings. I initially assumed that most therapists were empowered in this fashion but have discovered this is not true.

I think it is vitally important that training programs put more emphasis on how our early experiences may have determined both how we feel about ourselves and our patients and also how we think about the process. As Harris (2005) says, "Our blind spots arise from our own histories as well as our places in history and culture" (p. 275).

Another perspective on mutuality

It seems difficult for us to conceptualize mutuality as necessarily involving a degree of change and gratification for the analyst, though we may pay lip service to this idea. Both analyst and patient are motivated, ideally, to recreate our pasts with each other in the interests of making a difference that we couldn't make in childhood. The topic of the analyst's gratification should not be one of guilt and shame, but rather one of creative re-living. Again, that's why we have to treat people who we are interested in. If a patient cannot trigger an optimal degree of "positive transference" in us, we cannot significantly engage and help them at a deep level.

What interpersonal, relational, intersubjective, field theory, and mentalization all have in common is the recognition of psychoanalysis and psychotherapy not simply as a relationship but, if successful, one that necessarily involves a consistent mutual emotional engagement. This focus on the necessity of emotional engagement is perhaps the greatest change in not only analytic treatment but also in all forms of therapy. Goldfried and Davila (2005) note,

> As Gelso and Hayes (1998) have observed, the therapeutic relationship and technique "constantly interact with and influence one another. There is a profound synergism between the two. The techniques used by the therapists for example—and certainly the manner in which they are used—influence the kind of relationship that unfolds. Likewise, how the therapist feels toward the client will have a profound effect on the techniques he or she uses and the manner in which they are used with each client" (Gelso & Hayes, 1998, p. 8). Indeed, evidence exists to support this view. (p. 424)

The authors note that even Linehan, with her manualized responses to those with Borderline Personality Disorder, acknowledges that once a therapeutic alliance has been established, some degree of confrontation is needed. The therapist with manual in hand cannot avoid the conflict needed for change. In spite of the inevitability of bidirectional, ubiquitous communication, there remains the fiduciary responsibility to focus on the patient's needs over the analyst's, teasing out what is helpful and what is not. Movement toward new ways of being with patients has been painfully slow.

The analyst's ambivalence toward technique

In speaking to groups of therapists, I have noticed the palpable tension in the room when the topic of technique arises. The chief resistance to adopting technical guidelines often centers around a certain fear that therapists will lose the freedom to "be themselves," for lack of a better description. This perception that technique will rob them of their unique personalities, and the needs and desires they bring to treatment, creates an understandable resistance to even the most general suggestions of what works and what doesn't. Even the concept of technique often suggests some measure of artifice rather than creative spontaneity, even though this need not be the case.

I think this often means that therapists fear any interference with the path they need to take to either preserve or enhance themselves. Thus, the plurality of analytic theory and practice not only exemplifies the wide range of intellectual perspectives but also the need for analysts to resist any stance that might interfere with needed gratifications that could arise at any moment. At some level, they understand that they will necessarily play out their own early childhood dramas, as their patients play out theirs, and fear that adoption of technical guidelines will prevent them from doing so.

I think the following quote from Grossman (2014) illustrates what I am discussing.

> A theory of technique cast in terms of the analyst's behavior *is an effort to make the analyst's character disappear.* If it did so, we could teach analysis by teaching technique. But it does not work that way. A good analyst does not try to be someone else; he or she tries to use his or her strengths, receptivity, even the willingness to be wrong or blind or deaf at times, to good advantage. (p. 439, emphasis added)

I certainly agree that a good analyst does not try to be someone else. However, Grossman's view suggests an actual fear of psychic annihilation if any theory of technique is adopted. This type of fear of being so controlled as to be nonexistent no doubt also emanates from parallel experiences in childhood. But to what extent does this prevent us from seriously considering not just rigid technical prescriptions, but also any meaningful discussion of what might be an effective or ineffective type of intervention under similar circumstances? No current discussion of technique proposes hard and fast rules—only the possibility of technical guidelines. Nonetheless, as Fonagy (2003) has pointed out, "there are no new significant advances in technique" (p. 23). Some might argue that Fonagy's own work on mentalization does offer a new approach, and I would argue that my own work does as well.

I think if analysts in training were encouraged to be curious about what types of interventions seemed most comfortable and most uncomfortable for them, they might gain greater insight into how their own needs necessarily determine the how and why of their personal style, and they could then adapt them accordingly. As things stand now, interventions that have been accepted as inevitable and useful, like the judicious use of self-disclosure, remain controversial. Even in case reports that use self-disclosure to good advantage, the concluding advice usually focuses on disclaiming it as preferred intervention. Rather, the emphasis remains on the uniqueness of each analytic dyad, a topic I explore further in Chapter 5 on enactment.

As I have stated previously (Maroda, 1991, 2010), I think there is plenty of room for discovering general principles regarding interventions while allowing space for the analyst's individual style, personality, level of comfort, and even immediate need. No relationship, no matter how asymmetrical, can survive without some accommodation to the others' needs. The question I pursue in this volume is how we can incorporate a recognition and incorporation of our neediness into a model that retains a primary focus on helping the patient.

When young therapists ask me for advice on doing treatment, I tell them that they shouldn't treat anyone that they are not interested in. They can be ambivalent. But they can't really dislike the person at first meeting or have little or no interest in them. I also tell them to think hard about what they are feeling toward any prospective patient, what that patient needs to experience in treatment, and what they might need to get from that patient to make the relationship work. I emphasize conceptualizing the "match" (Kantrowitz, 1986, 2002) basically as a doable blending of the analyst's and patient's personalities (a topic I pursue in detail in Chapter 7). This usually includes some measure of shared early experience, no matter how different the analyst's and patient's lives appear to be. It goes without saying, of course, that all of this information is processed in the interests of creating the most effective focus on the patient's experience.

I think we need to have both pleasurable and unpleasurable experiences. The question is: Why is this idea of our role in the treatment process so controversial? Again, I think it reverts back to the fear of doing harm and the conviction that we need to martyr ourselves in order to do our job effectively and ethically. There is little to no room for conceiving some level of personal benefit for the therapist as normal, healthy, and inevitable, even though we all experience it on a regular basis. Nor is there much acknowledgement that we will also regularly feel boredom, disinterest, alienation, schadenfreude, anger, disgust, and shame.

Embracing our motivations

Embracing our early motivations for becoming therapists, especially our narcissistic needs and guilt, can help maximize the healthiest aspects of it in the treatment situation, and we can openly think and talk about how we need our patients. Acknowledging how this work helps us to find ourselves, maintain ourselves, and transform ourselves is essential to doing it well. I believe that both an overall examination of how and why we became therapists, what we as individuals are particularly looking for and gratified by in the process, and in what ways we are limited by biases formed in childhood could open up a whole new dialogue. That dialogue would include how our emotional responses can create new pathways for positively impacting our patients.

For example, a colleague who read this chapter noted that I am essentially challenging the therapists who I believe are too passive in their approach to the work, just as I challenged my mother's passivity.

I longed for her to be more proactive and, consequently, urge thera-pists to be more proactive. During my early adolescence, I became aware of my own passivity and worked hard to become more assertive. Admittedly, I overcorrected a bit, but then achieved more moderation as I worked through some of my defensiveness in my personal analysis.

However, once I began practicing from a traditional analytic stance, I became aware of how constrained I felt as a human being and even more aware of my patient's frustrations. I did not feel that I was adequately responding to them, but when I spoke to my analytic supervisors about this, I was told that this high level of frustration was a normal part of the process. I was urged to maintain my neu-trality. As I began my own treatment, I discovered that I also felt frustrated and blocked by my analyst's refusal to acknowledge her feelings and participation. One might say that overcoming passivity and the fear of acting has been a theme in my life and is therefore a theme in my development of theory and technique. Again, this does not mean that my views are either correct or incorrect, idiosyncratic or widely generalizable. It is for the reader to decide.

The analyst's persona

The analyst as arbiter of reality has been arguably replaced by the analyst as "good enough mother" who is more of a companion on the journey to self-awareness, seemingly not in possession of either the duty or the ability to direct the analytic process. Nowhere is this emphasis on "not knowing" more evident than in the current popularity of enactment (see Chapter 5). This does not mean that the analyst is not involved and working hard to understand the patient and the process; rather, it is a statement reflecting the move away from knowledge and authority to the elevated position of "not knowing." The elevation of "not knowing" emanates from the belief that we have a very limited capacity for awareness of either what we are feeling or what the patient is feeling. It is my position that what began as a laudable rejection of the analyst as all-knowing to a humbler awareness of our limitations has now become so all-encompassing that it discourages analysts from claiming any real knowledge or skill. (I say more about this in Chapter 7.) Mills (2017) argues for a more flexible approach to analytic knowledge and authority.

What perhaps appears to be the most widely shared claim in the relational tradition is the assault on the analyst's epistemological authority to objective knowledge … Why not say that knowledge is proportional or incremental rather than totalistic, thus subject to modification, alteration, and interpretation rather than categorically negate the category of an objective epistemology? Are there no objective facts? Would anyone care to defy the laws of gravity by attempting to fly off the roof of a building by flapping their arms? (pp. 316–317)

"Knowing" has become a synonym for arrogance and reductionism; "not knowing" presumes a more enlightened willingness to discover, an idea central to Buddhism. But this presumes that somehow what needs to surface will do so by virtue of this ongoing empathic stance. I have not found this to be true in my practice. Witnessing is valuable, but it is not enough. I find that although certain patients need very little direction and may even prefer to be left alone, many need ongoing gentle probing, interpretation, and confrontation.

The analyst as good object

An equally challenging concept centers on the idea that successful treatment depends on the analyst consistently being the badly needed good object in the patient's life. It is hard to argue the desirability of the analyst having qualities of empathy, patience, and a reasonable degree of kindness and good character. But as I discuss throughout this volume, "the analyst as good object" can foreclose or distort when held as an expectation. The idea of creating an opportunity where our patients can truly be free to discover themselves is probably closer to what most of us would actually subscribe to as an ideal. Yet, the impact of Winnicott's "good enough mother" proposition seems to have taken hold in a way that suggests a nurturing self-sacrificing stance that, to my mind, leaves little room for much working through of negative transference/countertransference emotions.

In spite of Winnicott's obvious intention in defining the mother's role in relation to the infant as necessarily imperfect yet "good enough," the adoption of his position to psychotherapists seems to have morphed into the "good enough" therapist being almost perfect. This may be due to the fact that Winnicott's case reports, particularly with regard to his psychoanalyst patient Margaret Little, centered on deviations from normal practice, including extended sessions, holding and stroking, and prophylactic hospitalization when he went on vacation. These "heroic" measures may have deliberately or inadvertently set the stage for defining "good enough" in terms of above and beyond the call. Perhaps this explains why the good enough mother persona appears routinely in current case reports, often emphasizing the analyst's unending kindness and willingness to sacrifice, rather than his or her skill. As Mendelsohn (2002) has pointed out,

> The therapist may try too hard to avoid mistakes or may feel obligated to take on the part of a new, good or contrasting object. These forms of avoidance and over conscientiousness may water down potential bad-enough experience, so that challenging analyst issues are only halfheartedly engaged. (p. 333)

In a recent edited volume of self-criticism by relational analysts, Mark (2018) discusses how there is increasingly only room for the "analyst's good-me" (p. 82).

Skovholt and Jennings (2004) make the point that unconscious, dysfunctional motives for becoming a therapist (e.g., voyeuristic tendencies, the need for power) can and do exist with altruistic and caring motives. The problem is not that we are secretly destructive or negative people pretending to be good. The problem is that we are so invested in being good and doing good for others that it is difficult for us to look at our normal human failings and desires. More importantly, this reluctance has been integrated into our theories, our persona, and our clinical preferences.

Buechler (2009) has spoken eloquently about our need for reparation and the tendency to be overly critical when we fail to meet the high standards we set for ourselves. She disagrees with Slochower's (2003) use of the terms "sins and delinquencies," fearing that this terminology only fuels the analyst's tendencies toward excessive guilt and shame. She makes a cogent argument for therapists to extend some of the same compassion to themselves that they extend to their patients, working on identifying repetitive countertransference patterns rather than identifying "sins."

I believe that when we are ashamed, as well as regretful, the strength we need to face our regrets may be sapped. Instead of being able to rise to the occasion of courageous self-confrontation, we feel shame's need to hide ourselves. It is impossible to simultaneously satisfy the essential tasks set by shame and regret. We may not be able to confront what we also deeply need to cover up. (p. 431)

I agree that shining the light of curiosity on our own behaviors, rather than negative judgment, ultimately leads to greater insight and responsibility.

The analyst's vulnerability

Arguably, classical analysts prided themselves on becoming the "bad objects," while relational analysts now pride themselves on being the good ones. Is our need to see ourselves as the "good mother" an unintended result of analysts no longer being able to write the patient's negative responses off as transference? Now that we believe in our own participation, it is harder to accept the patient's negative assessments without being too personally threatened or guilt-ridden.

Safran and Muran's (2002) expansion of Tronick's (1978, 1989) concept of rupture and repair may have inadvertently contributed to the popular notion that the therapeutic value of rupture resides in the analyst's willingness to assume responsibility for his or her participation and work quickly to restore peace (although this was not their intention). Many writers have questioned whether or not we are too quick to squash any conflict when it arises, even if it means placating a patient who is being unreasonable, in the belief that the therapeutic relationship will be damaged if we do not.

In reality, Safran and Muran (2002) said something quite different about countertransference and conflict.

Many therapeutic orientations assume that countertransference is at the heart of contemporary psychoanalytic technique. Despite this fact, systematic attempts to spell out the iterant processes involved in harnessing and working constructively with the intense, conflictual, and often painful feelings and thoughts that emerge for therapists when negotiating difficult moments with patients are rare. (p. 5)

As a young therapist reading the classical literature, I was consistently amazed at how frustrating classical analysts were and routinely viewed them as sadistically torturing their patients through a combination of unwanted interpretations, excessive silence, and refusing to acknowledge the patient's reality. Perhaps in the past we leaned more toward a sadistic provoking then closing down of the patient's anger. Do we now lean more toward a masochistic one that prevents it from surfacing? To me, these are two sides of the same dynamic.

Early career therapists often state that they feel like "frauds" because they are acutely aware of their anxiety, guilt, and shame over both their lack of knowledge and experience and their own neediness and problems. As much as the two-person movement has contributed greatly to understanding the analyst's flawed ongoing participation, there remains a therapeutic ideal wherein we assign ourselves the role of being, as one of my patients once described me, "perfectly human."

The therapist necessarily needs to achieve some degree of success in the pursuit of transforming the patient. In doing so, the analyst is affirmed and redeemed as she helps the patient. Patients who thwart us in our therapeutic aims (e.g., our desire to change them) quickly become the object of negative countertransference. Many treatments revolve around working through these miasmas. It sometimes feels as though a duel to the death is taking place, with each member of the analytic dyad determined to change the other. The best therapist for someone is the therapist who can most freely experience the patient's reality, as well as their own. That is why treating people we cannot emotionally engage with is both hopeless and unethical.

Given that some success is necessary, some degree of transformation, much of what is therapeutic for both patient and analyst is the mutual grieving of what cannot be. This can include the limits on individual change, the limits of the therapeutic relationship, and the limits of the analyst. There is always much to grieve.

Even though each therapist is unique, it still seems quite likely that we share many characteristics and childhood experiences, and I believe we naturally become frustrated and angry when our here-and-now efforts to transform our patients are thwarted. Correspondingly, we are equally gratified and relieved in an overdetermined fashion in those moments when we make a real difference. How might we behave and think differently if we were freer to acknowledge all of these feelings and needs? Pinsky (2011) wonders about the consequences of denying our human nature and says that the result of our denial is a form of self-idealization that threatens to erase both the analyst's and the patient's humanity and individual identity. Perhaps our image of "good enough" needs to be re-focused on authenticity rather than beneficence.

Hirsch (1997) has cited Searles' freedom to use his negative countertransference and character flaws to help his patients. Being uniquely in touch with his aforementioned realizations regarding his motivations for treating people appears to have freed him up to be more expressive and less ashamed of anger, frustration, and hatred: "Some analysts may feel unprofessional if, even privately, they acknowledge their own 'bad' feelings and thus need to fool themselves as well as try to hide them from their patients" (p. 257). Searles clearly did not have this problem. I think it is not a coincidence that Searles both had the ability to see himself as a guilty rescuer, based on early childhood experiences, and was also free to understand and use his negative feelings toward his patients rather than bury them. And perhaps this same self-awareness allowed him to love his patients with the abandon he describes, being gratified significantly in the course of doing treatment. He seems to have thought so when he said, "we need to become more freely *aware* of our omnipotent strivings, which are never 'resolved' throughout life and which remain, indeed, our most priceless wellspring of energy" (Searles, 1966, p. 33).

I believe there is insufficient dialogue regarding what fuels our beliefs and what determines our clinical choices. Psychoanalysis has situated itself firmly in the conceptualization of therapy as a relationship, acknowledging the analyst's contributions to that relationship. Yet, at the same time, there is almost no discussion of *why* we have forged a new relational perspective that emphasizes the patient's early deficits, trauma, and even fragility, or why therapeutic action increasingly focuses on what we don't know versus what we do.

Theory is personal

How much of what we do in the clinical hour satisfies our own needs, and how much of psychoanalytic theory is based on the shared early experience of those who chose this profession? Daniel Jacobs (2000) says that each person's theory is "a subjective one based on the inner interpersonal world of the theorist ... which may explain why attachment to particular theories may be so intense and why debate over theory has, at times, become so acrimonious" (p. 307). In essence, Jacobs tells us that we each have created a theory that is *essentially about ourselves.* And perhaps that is why arguments about theory can become so heated and personal. If you negate my theory, are you then negating me? And can understanding just how personal our theories can be also help us to step back and be more open to alternate views? Kite (2016) notes that "many of us remain bewildered as to *why we became analysts in the first place,* and become 'experts' in this or that, either as an effort to cover ourselves or to have an authoritative voice" (p. 1156).

Although the inevitable personal nature of our theories may make us overly enamored with them or overly defensive when they are challenged, one could easily argue that theories of anything are born out of some thinker's early experience. The fact that theories are personal certainly does not discredit them; they are simply our views of the world. Using our own perspectives to create theory is creative and productive, and from my perspective, those who possess the intellectual fortitude to think out their positions and publish them have something valuable to contribute to the dialogue, even if you disagree with them on many fronts. Greater recognition of the personal nature of our theories might well allow us to not only be more respectful toward those we disagree with but also humbler when presenting our own ideas. Understanding this personal authorship of theory and technique naturally lends itself to more scrutiny. As McWilliams (2004) observes,

> I have concluded over the years that when clinicians talk most passionately about an attitude or process that is "at the center of" or that is "the essence of" the healing process, they often prescribe a stance that either normalized their own dispositions or compensates for the limitations of their character type. (p. 148)

Again, this does mean we need to discount any theory simply because it is personal. I have said previously our theories are only more likely to be highly idiosyncratic if our childhood has been as well (Maroda, 1991). The more similar we are to others, the more generalizable our theories will be.

We do not generally ask how our childhood experiences generated both theory and practice, even though we give lip service to the idea that our theories have been based, in large part, by the personalities of the people who created them (e.g., Benjamin, 2010; Bromberg & Aron, 2019; Cooper, 1986; Harris, 1998; Stolorow & Atwood, 1979) and the cultural context of the time. Jacobs (1993), citing Kohut's lonely childhood and subsequent keen appreciation and need for empathy, says we rarely make this obvious connection from early experience to theory: "Because we do not expect a high degree of self-revelation at public meetings or in our literature, this tie of theory to our own early relationships often goes unmentioned" (p. 309). Steinberg (2016) echoes these sentiments: "The analysts' deeply held and deeply personal desires for particular experiences with their patients ... become clothed in essentialist notions of the psychoanalytic process" (pp. 72–73).

The transition from classical to relational analysis

The two-person approaches to psychoanalysis were created by my generation, all of us having experienced the dark side of neutrality and abstinence and knowing that there had to be a better way. Suffice it to say, a paradigm shift toward a less authoritarian, more empathic, and more mutual way of seeing people and doing treatment was in full force. And the older, outdated views of how the analyst-patient dyad interacted have largely fallen away.

The questions that I think we have not adequately pursued are these: How did classical analysis become a caricature of itself, often resulting in excessive thwarting and frustrating of patients; how were we able to free ourselves of those constraints and create something new; and how might we have gone astray in our attempts to humanize and elevate the analytic process? If we have, in fact, overcorrected, then what is the path to free ourselves from this impasse? What common factors are operative in the creation of analytic theory and practice, ranging from the classical analysis to modern day relational, interpersonal, and intersubjective theories that limit our creativity and capacity for self-awareness?

In spite of the relational, interpersonal, and intersubjective turns of the last three decades, emphasizing the ubiquity of counter-transference, the fallibility of the therapist, and the inevitable mutuality and co-construction of the therapeutic relationship, it seems to me that we have retained the perfectionistic aspects of the past in our current persona. Inspired by dramatic case presentations where the modern two-person analyst pulls the intuition-based perfect intervention out of the hat, it seems to me that, in spite of our claims for imperfection and fallibility, our self-depictions convey a pursuit of empathic, here-and-now responding that is beyond illusive. It is perfection. As Pinsky (2011) notes, "The myth of the fully analyzed analyst, far from disappearing, lives on in conceptions of the analyst with superhuman capacity to do the demanding work" (p. 367).

Have we not replaced the all-knowing, perfectly analyzed, and objective Freudian analyst with the aforementioned good mother with infinite patience and the capacity for "holding" the patient's experience? Have we eschewed the image of the authoritarian, all-knowing analyst in favor of the all-beneficent good mother? Noting the considerable change in perspective over the past 40 years, Levenson (2009) observes,

> The current emphasis on the vicissitudes of early mothering, especially as described in attachment theory, reflects a cultural change, from the patriarchal, oedipal-oriented (conflict and envy) world in which I both grew up and became an analyst, to a matriarchal, nurturing one in which early mothering and empathy are privileged. (p. 163)

Levenson's point illustrates the changes that occur across generations and evolving culture. During the period when he was trained, most psychoanalysts in American were white, Jewish physicians; women had not yet made a real dent in the professional world. It was, indeed, a traditional male's world.

The classic approach for creating neutrality among the American medical analysts was anchored in the illusion that, having been analyzed themselves, these analysts (who were overwhelmingly male physicians) were essentially "cured" of their need to heal themselves through being an analyst. Their authoritarian, "everything-as-transference" approach allowed them to believe that no matter how severely they might be criticized by their patients, it was really their patients' anger at their mothers that was at the heart of their despair. The analyst was essentially a neutral and, more importantly, *innocent bystander in the replaying of the patient's early experiences.*

After generations of people were analyzed and expressed dissatisfaction with the results—some even feeling that they had been abused and taken for their money—we witnessed the rise of behaviorism. Psychoanalysis began to fall out of favor, often being derided by psychology professors at major universities. Soon they would be joined by psychiatry, emphasizing the usefulness of psychotropic drugs over talk therapy. The judgment was in: Psychoanalysts had failed to put their patients' well-being ahead of their own, in spite of elaborate theoretical and clinical rationales they developed to justify their behavior. Their form of treatment was considered ineffective and wasteful at best and fraudulent at worst.

Societal factors, especially the post-Vietnam War era, brought widespread rejection of arbitrary authority, resulting in greater skepticism about analytic treatment. It also brought reductions in insurance coverage as managed care emerged, seizing on reducing mental health benefits for quick profits. Another huge change was soon to take place—the American Psychological Association's 1988 lawsuit against the American Psychoanalytic Association (APsaA) for unfair restraint of trade. The basis for the legal action was APsaA's exclusion of all but physicians for analytic training at their institutes, as well as decades of public statements about how their incomes would be negatively impacted if other mental health professionals could become analysts. The courts ruled in favor of the four psychologists who brought the suit, and damages were paid by APsaA, along with removing the physician requirement for analytic training.

So how is this historical information relevant to my thesis? It marked the beginning of a significant change in the make-up and background of psychoanalytic trainees. I propose that the influx of social workers and psychologists, with their liberal arts backgrounds and different personality styles, contributed significantly to generating the two-person approach. Our theories began to change because the people creating them were different. Not only did they have different backgrounds and education than the psychiatrists who preceded them, they increasingly were female rather than male. Even if men were still doing most of the publishing, the influence of women was undeniable. Women have now outnumbered men in the ranks of psychoanalysts, and their influence regarding the adoption of attachment theory and a "holding environment" are self-evident.

The majority of psychoanalysts today are female non-physicians. Though still mostly White, they actively recruit minority representation and embrace multiculturism. A look at the programs of all analytic conferences over the last 20 years reveals a remarkable shift in perspective, focusing heavily on culture, gender, race, and class. There is little doubt that societal changes, as well as the education and gender of psychoanalysts, has deeply affected our theoretical and clinical choices. Yet, if our shared motivations for becoming analysts have not changed, then there must remain a common thread that runs through these changes. I believe that common thread is the aforementioned guilt, the need for redemption, and the inevitable frustrations and gratifications that arise.

We have made huge progress in acknowledging what, to date, is the single most important determinant of treatment outcome—the therapeutic relationship. We have all benefited greatly from the humanizing effect of evolving perspectives on the nature of therapist patient relationship. Relational theory critic Jon Mills (2005) credits relational theory for having contributed greatly to freeing up analysts to be more expressive and present.

Yet at the same time, relational theory has arguably become rigid in its views. Even those who purport to encourage collegial debate rarely challenge other in-group members' opinions or interventions. Journal and online commentaries typically do little more than confirm the main author's or panelist's positions. References are almost always restricted to other in-group members' work, and the terms "rich," "beautifully written," and "courageous" are bandied about so often as to be rendered meaningless. I fear that we are moving toward replacing self-scrutiny with self-congratulation. We rarely examine painful aspects of our participation in the therapeutic endeavor and in our profession. The contributors to *De-Idealizing Relational Theory: A Critique from Within* (Aron et al., 2018) recognized and attempted to correct this problem, but I think more incorporation of critiques from those who are not part of the inner circle would be beneficial. In-group members can only be so critical of their close colleagues. More constructive criticisms and questioning among all of the different theoretical schools of thought, as Stephen Mitchell envisioned when he created *Psychoanalytic Dialogues*, could go a long way in furthering our creativity. Bearing in mind the personal nature of our theoretical stances, along with the shared, overdetermined nature of our vocational choice, could help us bear witness not only to our patients, but to each other.

Conclusion

Psychoanalytic theory and practice have been forged over the past century by the individuals and the culture from which they came. More critical to understanding theory and practice and to their creative evolvement is the acceptance of the ongoing basis for them both in the individual and collective psyches of the people who create them. Our personal motivations for being analysts and theorists naturally arise from our own childhood experiences. Our explanations of the world are also explanations of ourselves. And only the fullest possible self-awareness of these experiences and our resulting needs can facilitate the evolution of analytic theory and technique.

In this chapter, I have attempted to set the stage for the rest of this volume, which will contain further elaborations on the notions of our personal attributes, early experiences, and vulnerabilities lying at the heart of analytic theory and practice. I invite the reader on this journey with me.

References

Aron, L., Grand, S., & Slochower, J. (Eds.) (2018). *De-idealizing relational theory: A critique from within*. New York: Routledge.

Benjamin, J. (2010). Where's the gap and what's the difference? The relational view of intersubjectivity, multiple selves, and enactment. *Contemporary Psychoanalysis, 46*, 112–119.

Brenner, C. (1985). Countertransference as a compromise formation. *Psychoanalytic Quarterly, 54*, 155–163.

Bromberg, P., & Aron, L. (2019). Disguised autobiography as clinical case study. *Psychoanalytic Dialogues, 29*, 695–710.

Buechler, S. (2009). The analyst's search for atonement. *Psychoanalytic Inquiry*, *29*, 426–436.

Celenza, A. (2010). The analyst's need and desire. *Psychoanalytic Dialogues*, *20*, 60–69.

Cooper, A. (1986). Some limitations on therapeutic effectiveness: The "burn out" syndrome. *Psychoanalytic Quarterly*, *55*, 576–598.

Fonagy, P. (2003). Some complexities in the relationship of psychoanalytic theory to technique. *Psychoanalytic Quarterly*, *72*, 13–47.

Gerson, M.J. (2018). Death of a parent: Openings at an ending. *Psychoanalytic Perspectives*, *15*, 340–354.

Goldfried, M., & Davila, J. (2005). The role of relationship and technique in therapeutic change. *Psychotherapy: Theory, Research, Practice, Training*, *4*, 421–430.

Grossman, L. (2014). Analytic technique: A reconsideration of the concept. *Psychoanalytic Review*, *101*, 431–449.

Harris, A. (1998). The analyst as (auto)biographer. *American Imago*, *55*, 255–275.

Harris, A. (2005). Conflict in relational treatments. *Psychoanalytic Quarterly*, *74*, 267–293.

Hirsch, I. (1997). Analytic intimacy, analyzability, and the vulnerable analyst. *Free Associations*, *7*, 250–259.

Jacobs, D. (2000). Theory and its relation to early affective experience. In S. L. Ablon, D. Brown, E. J. Khantzian, & J. E. Mack (Eds.), *Human Feelings: Explorations in affect development and meaning* (pp. 305–316). Hillsdale, NJ: The Analytic Press.

Jacobs, T. J. (1993). The inner experiences of the analyst: Their contribution to the analytic process. *International Journal of Psychoanalysis*, *74*, 7–14.

Kantrowitz, J. L. (1986). The role of the patient-analyst "match" in the outcome of psychoanalysis. *Annals of Psychoanalysis*, *14*, 273–297.

Kantrowitz, J. L. (2002). The triadic match: The interactive effect of supervisor, candidate, and patient. *Journal of the American Psychoanalytic Association*, *50*, 939–968.

Kite, J. V. (2016). The fundamental ethical ambiguity of the analyst as a person. *Journal of the American Psychoanalytic Association*, *64*, 1153–1171.

Kravis, N. (2013). The analyst's hatred of analysis. *Psychoanalytic Quarterly*, *82*, 89–114.

Levenson, E. A. (2009). The enigma of the transference. *Contemporary Psychoanalysis*, *45*, 163–178.

Luchner, A. F., Mose, C. J., Mirsalimi, H., & Jones, R. A. (2008). Maintaining boundaries in psychotherapy: Covert narcissistic personality characteristics and psychotherapists. *Psychotherapy, Theory, Research, Practice, Training*, *45*, 1–14.

Mark, D. (2018). Forms of equality in relational psychoanalysis. In L. Aron, S. Grand, & J. Slochower, J. (Eds.), *De-idealizing relational theory: A critique from within* (pp. 80–101). New York: Routledge.

Maroda, K. (1991). *The power of countertransference: Innovations in analytic technique*. Chichester, UK: Wiley.

Maroda, K. (2010). *Psychodynamic techniques: Working with emotion in the therapeutic relationship*. New York: Guilford.

McWilliams, N. (2004). *Psychoanalytic psychotherapy: A practitioner's guide*. New York: Guilford.

Mendelsohn, E. (2002). The analyst's bad-enough participation. *Psychoanalytic Dialogues*, *12*, 331–358.

Miller, A. (1997). *The drama of the gifted child: The search for the true self*. New York: Basic Books.

Mills, J. (2005). A critique of relational psychoanalysis. *Psychoanalytic Psychology*, *22*, 155–188.

Mills, J. (2017). Challenging relational psychoanalysis: A critique of post-modernism and analyst self-disclosure. *Psychoanalytic Perspectives*, *14*, 313–335.

Olinick, S. L. (1980). *The psychotherapeutic instrument*. New York: Jason Aronson.

Orange, D. (2016). *Nourishing the life of clinicians and humanitarians: The ethical turn in psychoanalysis*. New York: Routledge.

Pinsky, E. (2011). The Olympian delusion. *Journal of the American Psychoanalytic Association*, *59*, 351–375.

Prodgers, A. (1991). On hating the patient. *British Journal of Psychotherapy*, *8*, 144-154.

Safran, J., & Muran, J. C. (2002). *Negotiating the therapeutic alliance*. New York: Guilford.

Searles, H. F. (1966). Feelings of guilt in the psychoanalyst. *Psychiatry*, *29*, 319–323.

Searles, H. F. (1979). *Countertransference and related subjects*. New York: International Universities Press.

Skovholt, T. M., & Jennings, L. (2004). *Master therapist: Exploring expertise in therapy and counseling*. Boston: Allyn & Bacon.

Slochower, J. (2003). The analyst's secret delinquencies. *Psychoanalytic Dialogues*, *13*, 45–469.

Steinberg, B. (2016). How much needs to change in analysis. How do we get there? *Journal of the American Psychoanalytic Association*, *64*, 177–192.

Stolorow, R., & Atwood, G. (1979). *Faces in a cloud: Subjectivity in personality theory*. Northvale, NJ: Jason Aronson.

Storr, A. (1979). *The art of psychotherapy*. London: Secker and Warburg.

Sussman, M. (1992). *A curious calling*. New York: Jason Aronson.

Tronick, E. Z. (1989). Emotions and emotional communications in infants. *American Psychologist, 44*, 112–119.

Tronick, E. Z., Als, H., Adamson, L., Wise, S., & Brazelton, T. B. (1978). The infant's response to entrapment between contradictory messages in face-to-face interaction. *Journal of the American Academy of Child Psychiatry, 17*, 1–13.

Wachtel, P. (2007). *Relational theory and the practice of psychotherapy*. New York: Guilford Press.

Chapter 2

Managing the analyst's needs

To what extent does the analyst need to renounce his or her own needs in the interests of serving the patient? And to what extent does the analyst need to be gratified by or somehow benefit from the relationship with the patient in order for the treatment to progress and succeed? The dialectic between gratification and renunciation is both a familiar one, yet also an ill-defined and perplexing one. We know that we do sacrifice for our patients. But we also know that we are deeply gratified by our relationships with them. The goal of this chapter is to review and integrate the literature on sacrifice and gratification, with an eye toward greater understanding of both what we give and what we receive in the context of doing treatment. I also want to illustrate how relative those concepts can be both within and across individuals, depending on current emotional state, relationship status, physical well-being, and developmental stages.

Suffice it to say that the notion of our self-sacrifice gleans far more positive attention than the topic of our gratification and/or our enduring personal benefit resulting directly from doing treatment. Perhaps those who so strongly oppose the idea of therapist gratification do so out of fear that the needed ethic of discipline, patience, and self-sacrifice may be undermined or even forfeited once gratification is accepted. Yet, all close human relationships necessarily involve a high degree of both sacrifice and gratification.

The idea that these two concepts cannot coexist within the parameters of the therapeutic dyad is counterintuitive. Yes, a higher degree of focus on the other person, and the ability to quietly listen and accept his or her pain, is part of what distinguishes us from friends, family, and other potential listeners. Rather than jumping in with our own stories or rushing to find a solution, we often earn our fees through a sometimes torturous process of silent witnessing. Yet, this is not the whole story.

The therapeutic relationship provides ample room for both healthy self-sacrifice and healthy, mutually beneficial gratification. Unhealthy sacrifice and gratification also exist, of course. Sacrifice sometimes leads to deep resentment and an uncomfortable sense of having submitted to a sadistic patient, while at other times it brings the tranquil satisfaction of having relinquished pride and power in the interests of another. Similarly, gratification, particularly the currently sanctioned activity of "play" in the analytic encounter, can be easily enjoyed and accepted. But feeling loved, deeply understood, found attractive, or taken care of, particularly at a vulnerable moment in the analyst's life, may promote guilt or even shame. How are we to discern when our needs are being met in the interests of the patient or at his or her expense? And when does healthy self-sacrifice devolve into masochistic submission?

The greatest obstacle to integrating these two ways of being is the erroneous assumption that ongoing personal gratification of the analyst's needs is automatically at odds with doing right by the patient. Unraveling this dilemma is highly dependent on accepted definitions of self-interest, benefit, and gratification. Self-indulgence has unfortunately often been seen as an inevitable consequence of accepting self-interest, particularly in a formal way. Again, there is a measure of distrust and fear of doing harm when the topic of analyst self-interest arises. As Sussman (1992) states,

> The simple truth is that each practitioner possesses a unique constellation of motives for practice—some altruistic, others grounded more deeply in self-interest. Shapiro and Gabbard (1994) point out that an excess of either narcissistic gratification or selfless devotion can have detrimental effects on treatment outcome. Therefore, they add, it's time to move beyond a moralistic notion of "good" or "bad." Only the optimal balance of both can provide an adequate foundation for effective psychotherapy. (p. xvii)

Keep in mind that Sussman's statements are from 1992. The absence of any real dialogue on this topic says much about our openness to these ideas. We avoid discussions of what is reasonable and what is not, for fear that we will appear to be endorsing exploitation and indulgence clothed as self-preservation. When I talk about the analyst's inevitable self-interest, I am not talking about sexual gratification, stock tips, excessive idealization, and the like. To be clear, I am talking about the give and take and mutual acknowledgement that are part and parcel of any human relationship. This dynamic that can, and does, exist within the ethical boundaries of a professional therapeutic relationship appropriately focused on the patient. Coen (2000) discusses the pervasive fear of openly admitting to our wishes and fears.

> At conferences and in discussion groups, some colleagues seem excessively fearful of the "slippery slope" of analysts' wishes and feelings. This superego-ish attitude seems intended to rein in the rest of us, as if we were at imminent risk of enacting our wishes and feelings with our patients. I have reassured these colleagues that I do not act on my wishes and feelings toward my patients; rather, as I attend to my patients, I continually scan my inner experience, for the sake of their analyses. Such reassurance has not calmed these colleagues' concerns about inappropriate action. Yet we share the conviction that our best protection against such action is maximum responsibility for our needs, wishes, desires, and feelings toward our analysands. (pp. 804–805)

I think the operative phrase in Coen's remarks is that benefit accrues to him *as he attends to his patients*. The idea of analysts prioritizing their own needs over their patients, although this does happen in the real world, is essentially a straw man when discussing the realities of everyday practice. It is also another expression of the pervasive distrusts of self and/or others and the aforementioned fear of harming the patient. Ironically, our reluctance to look hard at our own needs and how they might be met constructively hampers our efforts to know when we are doing so *unconstructively*. We cannot possibly assess the impact of our interventions if we are unwilling or unable to examine our own neediness.

The literature on both the analyst's sacrifice and gratification or benefit is so sparse as to be almost nonexistent. More private and public conversation on this continuum from sacrifice to gratification is required for adequate insight and to adequately prepare clinicians for the emotional roller coaster they will experience, especially as they begin their careers. The difficulty of the subject is not sufficient reason to ignore it, particularly when it is often the proverbial elephant in the consulting room.

I am sympathetic to how relative our personal needs and our capacity for being emotionally generous may be at any given time. I am also sympathetic to the notion that what we can, or even should, give or not give at any point in time is highly dependent on what the patient can tolerate. Yet without an ongoing professional dialogue on these matters, we are essentially left with our own private decisions—ones that are too often guided by fear, guilt, and shame. When in doubt, clinicians tend to err on the side of being overly passive and submissive. When working with a difficult patient, a vicious cycle of masochistic submission, followed by resentment and withdrawal or even punishment, followed by guilt and shame-based further sacrifice, can easily take hold. This cycle is quite evident in reading case examples centered on long-lasting impasses. Unfortunately, the resolution of these impasses is rarely described as resulting in new insight on the analyst's part. Rather, we have become resigned to the position of not knowing, with resolution being too often dependent on enactment.

The sparse literature on our own gratification includes Michael Shulman's (2016) article on "unavoidable satisfactions," where he focuses on the unique opportunities afforded to analysts for incomparable hour-to-hour and day-to-day intimacy with others that is unparalleled. He also laments that while we may intellectually accept the inevitable gratifications of the analyst, we choose not to openly discuss it. Rosenblatt (2009) calls for both open discussion and formal research on the topic of gratification. This chapter examines both self-sacrifice and gratification, aiming to balance these two vital aspects of our work. The following vignette illustrates what I believe to be commonplace therapist behavior.

I attended a retirement party for a therapist a few years ago who was respected and well-liked in the therapist community. Her adult son stood up and did a rather amusing monologue about what it was like to grow up with a therapist mother. Although he was clearly proud of his mother and loved her very much, he ambivalently re-called stories of family dinners routinely being interrupted by patients calling their home phone directly. He reminded the audience that when he was a boy all phones had cords, so his mother would leave the dinner table, go to the phone nearest the bathroom, then extend the phone around into the bathroom and close the door.

She would often stay on the phone for an hour with a patient in distress. During this time the family could not use what was then the only bathroom. They ate dinner with their wife and mother absent from the table, had to speak in hushed voices, then had to move around the house by sneaking under or over the outstretched phone cord. Everyone in the audience laughed at this story and was moved by the son's recounting of his mother's devotion. And I laughed as hard as anyone.

But I also found myself thinking how totally unnecessary these calls were and how they met this woman's need to be needed in a profound and primitive way that could not be gratified by her family and many friends. I want to add that even as a young therapist I found these stories of "self-sacrifice" common even among classical analysts presenting their patients at conferences.

I recall my confusion when classical analysts who wrote about abstinence and neutrality also recounted giving out their home phone numbers, taking calls in the middle of the night, and both calling and writing to patients while on vacation. More notably, they did not discuss these behaviors as aberrations or breaks in the therapeutic frame. Rather, they were presented as part and parcel of being an analyst or, conversely, as a thinly disguised expression of their noble selflessness.

We currently see a revival of this need to be needed in therapists giving out their private cell phone numbers and texting with patients at all hours of the day and night. These very same therapists will say that it is unseemly for a therapist to have his or her needs met by a patient on a regularly basis. My point here is that one of the un-intended consequences of not admitting, even to ourselves, how much we need from our patients, often results in enabling behaviors rivaling Winnicott's prophylactic hospitalization of his patients. I believe we need to find more productive ways to have our deep needs to be needed met. This cannot happen, of course, until we openly acknowledge that we have needs that have to be met in order for us to continue our work. It is my contention that therapist overcompensations and pathological enactments have been essentially institutionalized over time, regardless of theoretical orientation, fueled by this denial of our needs.

Levinas and the analyst as self-sacrificing

As we eschew the concept of analyst gratification, it is not surprising that the pendulum has swung in quite the opposite direction. The work of French philosopher Emmanuel Levinas has become increasingly popular in analytic circles as we debate the value and necessity of the analyst's position as "sacrificing other." Briefly, Levinas, a survivor of a Nazi labor camp, maintains that we all have an ethical obligation to sacrifice for others, to the put the *other's* need ahead of our own in an act of *radical responsibility*. Reflecting on Levinas's philosophy, Alford (2000) describes Levinas's theory, wherein Levinas himself openly admits that it goes against our nature to relinquish self-interest. Nonetheless, his ethical stance is one that compels us to do exactly what I discourage—attempting to transcend human nature: "'Ethics is, therefore, *against nature* because it forbids the murderousness of my natural will to put my own existence first' (Levinas, 1986, p. 24, emphasis in original). All that is ethical about humans stems from their transcendence of nature" (p. 249).

Relying on transcendence and constant sacrifice as an ethical stance in daily living seems self-evidently impossible to me. How can this stance be realistically integrated into a viable context for analytic treatment? Donna Orange (2016b) has attempted to integrate Levinas's views into the clinical practice of psychoanalysis, focusing on the interpersonal implications of his work. Flowing from her previous work on emotion (Orange, 1995), she makes a compelling and passionate plea for the analyst's vulnerability and surrender to the patient's experience (she builds on the work of Ghent and Levinas in their depictions of what might be called "healthy suffering" that is, at its essence, shared emotional pain, even though the stated objective is mutual vulnerability). I find this idea compelling, filled with tenderness and a spiritual/philosophical property of transcendence.

Nonetheless, simply by invoking Levinas, whose philosophy arguably ventures beyond the limits of healthy suffering, invites comparisons to masochism. Regarding Levinas's central position of *infinite responsibility for other*, Orange (2016a) readily acknowledges this raises the scepter of moral masochism. Her reply is, "Please read Manny Ghent" (p. 58)—a reference to Ghent's (1990) classic article on distinguishing between emotional surrender and masochistic submission. Orange's point, of course, is that following Levinas's philosophy for the purpose of facilitating emotional surrender is substantively the opposite of masochism.

Given my own work on mutual emotional surrender (Maroda, 1999), I cannot argue with the wisdom of facilitating it, as well as agreeing that a degree of selflessness is involved in doing so. However, the notion of *infinite responsibility* for others does not sit well with me, echoing what I have described previously in this volume as the residue of the analyst's childhood, guilt-based burden. I don't believe that mutual emotional surrender requires the degree of self-sacrifice or the extreme asymmetry described by Levinas and Orange. Even though Orange (2016a) encourages clinicians to be aware of the dangers of falling into masochistic submission, she admits this can be difficult to discern.

> Are we simply, in our welcoming response to the other—especially when it stretches us, as working in the service of the other often must—living out unanalyzed moral masochism? Should we be setting better limits, for our own sakes and—as many theorists would argue—for that of the patent as well? Better limits according to whom? How do we decide which phone call not to take, which extra session to refuse, which patient not to take? How do we decide what is service to the other, and what is masochism? (p. 63)

To my mind, these questions already suggest some degree of masochistic submission. In the same volume, Orange pointed out that we need to avoid the neophyte's common mistake of taking patients we cannot successfully engage with and to avoid depleting ourselves. Yet this quote suggests that she struggles with not treating certain people and turning down requests from patients that may be unreasonable. I say this not to criticize Orange, whose work I admire and cite, but rather to demonstrate my point about how our personal struggles with being responsible for other's pain is evidenced in our theories and practice.

When I read her words, "I do not *become* my brother's keeper. I am born into that responsibility; I may evade it, but it's always already mine" (p. 138), I couldn't help but think of the therapist's guilty responsibility for others that begins so early it is hard to remember a time when it did not exist. On a personal level, I am inspired by Orange's overall emphasis on morality and ethics. And I cannot argue with the idea that we can do more as clinicians than we have in the past. But I can argue with the notion that the path to greater effectiveness and, if you will, to the greater good lies primarily in sacrifice. It has been my contention for decades that while empathy, kindness, and establishing a safe environment are essential, it is *compassionate authenticity*, rather than *infinite responsibility*, that we must struggle to achieve.

Rather than emphasizing authenticity, we are increasingly defining our role as a self-sacrificing one, perhaps in a vain attempt to erase our awareness of our neediness and vulnerability. Just as with our preoccupation with being the "good object," we run the risk of further distorting the analytic persona with these unrealistic attributes. Over time, of course, these distortions come to define us, creating and re-creating an analytic ideal that denies our humanity and, as I stated in the previous chapter, perpetuates a vision of us as perfect. An emphasis on sacrifice in the literature naturally produces clinical practice that mirrors it. Akhtar and Varma (2012) discussed this concept in terms of cultural norms, noting that once sacrifice is incorporated into the language of a people, it becomes a shared reverence and part of a shared cultural psyche. I think this applies to the analytic culture as well.

I might add that arguments for us being akin to humanitarians runs the risk of furthering our analytic ideal of unconditional acceptance of our patients and silently suffering to make them well. It reimagines us as bordering on sainthood if we do our job well. What is notably lacking in this conversation is the stress and negative emotions that also accompany analytic work. As Kravis (2013) points out,

Some analysts speak of analytic work with a kind of spiritual rapture. There is certainly a place for pleasure and pride in the triumphs of analytic work, as long as there is room also for feeling sick and tired of it, exhausted or bored by it, frustrated and disappointed with it. (p. 108)

Pinsky (2011) examines what she sees as the negative consequences of a potential idealized selfless analyst persona, implying the result is a merger that threatens the essential boundaries.

The more the therapist believes in a heroic capacity for selfless service to the patient, and the more he is conceptualized as above being a subject himself, the greater the danger of erasing the line that keeps the patient safe. Where there is only one entity, there can be no separation. (p. 368)

How might we best conceptualize the needed degree and type of sacrifice in analytic work? Because of the lack of formal discussion of this topic as it pertains to psychotherapy, I turned to the social psychology literature in hopes of finding some research results that might apply to the therapeutic dyad.

The literature on sacrifice in close relationships

The literature on close relationships, which focuses on intimate partners rather than therapists, friends, or other types of close relationships, cannot be legitimately generalized to the analytic relationship. Yet I believe it does offer some insights worthy of consideration. It has long been established that good therapeutic relationships begin with trust, genuineness, and empathy. But the research on close relationships offer some additional information that we might productively use. On the issue of self-sacrifice, Van Lange et al. (1997) state that,

In the context of ongoing, close relationships, *willingness to sacrifice*, is defined as the propensity to forego immediate self-interest to promote the well-being of a partner or relationship. Sacrifice may entail the forfeiting of behaviors that might otherwise be desirable, enacting of behaviors that might otherwise be undesirable, or both. (pp. 1373–1374)

At first glance, this research seems to confirm the centrality of self-sacrifice in good close relationships. And it does—but there is more to add. As it turns out, the motivation for the self-sacrifice is critical to its consequences for both parties involved. When a person sacrifices out of a genuine desire to please the other, the outcome for both is generally positive. However, when one person sacrifices out of a desire to avoid conflict or some other negative response, the outcome is equally negative. Impett et al. (2005) defined these two basic categories as *approach motives* versus *avoidance motives*. They discuss how vitally important the motivation for sacrifice is to the outcome.

[G]ratifying a partner's wishes to make him or her happy (an approach motive) may lead to increased pleasure and positive emotions through the process of empathic identification (e.g., Blau, 1964; Lerner et al., 1976). However, sacrificing to prevent conflict (an avoidance motive) may at best lead to relief and at worst produce the very anxiety and tension that individual was trying to avoid (Downey et al., 1998). (p. 129)

Righetti and Impett (2017) state further that "suppressing one's genuine feelings when making a sacrifice is typically costly for both partners in relationships" (p. 4).

In addition, level of commitment has been identified as a vitally important component of satisfying self-sacrifice. The more committed individuals are to the relationship, the more likely they are to sacrifice based on a healthy approach motive. The greater their fear of rejection, the more likely they were to sacrifice based on an avoidance motive. I think there are two potential inferences for the therapy relationship we might consider. One, it seems that some people are much more prone to enjoying making another person happy, even if this requires ongoing sacrifice. Thus, some therapists could reasonably sacrifice more than others and would be better suited to treat patients who require it. Second, therapists with insecure attachment style might well fall into masochistic, conflict-avoidant sacrifices based on fear of rejection and loss. Again, I

believe that the issues like these could be brought up for consideration in analytic and other training programs, thus facilitating greater
insight regarding our motivations for certain behaviors and greater
consideration of who we can work well with.

In addition to pondering our general styles of relations, it may well
be the case that the motives, even for the same therapist, might differ
at different times and with different patients. It would seem that
intention, which I will take up later in this volume, speaks volumes in
terms of results. Our tolerances vary from day to day, or even from
hour to hour. And, as stated previously, our level of caring and
commitment to a particular patient also affects what we have to give,
whether we like that idea or not.

The basic notions of commitment, caring, security, and emotional
honesty being critical to the success or failure of any self-sacrificial
act in close relationships seems so fundamental I doubt that similar
examinations of long-term analytic relationships would yield sub-
stantially different results. Impett et al. (2005) also simply state that
what is in one person's best interest is ultimately also in the other's.

This notion of mutuality in close relationships squares with my
own long-time conviction that mutuality is the order of the day in any
ongoing close relationship. The theory of mutuality dictates that
anything that is good for the patient (good meaning constructive and
healthy over the long term) is ultimately good for the analyst and vice
versa. (This is in contrast to what may feel good or be gratifying in
the moment.) Gabbard (1995) and Celenza (2007) have repeatedly
confirmed that what we consider to be the worst self-indulgences at
the patient's expense (e.g., sexual and other significant boundary
violations) necessarily produce painful consequences for both therapist and patient. Likewise, growth-promoting transformative experiences for the patient necessarily produce some level of transformation
for the analyst.

Before moving on to the topic of the analyst's gratification and
benefits from doing treatment, I want to say more about the implications of *approach motives* and how they are both relatively dis-
tributed among individuals, and also how they are integral to the
group identity of both analysts and therapists in general. We all have
different tolerances, not to mention that our level of tolerance changes
with both our immediate and our developmental circumstances. But

we need to also hold some concept of generally acceptable and healthy boundaries and degree of sacrifice. If we sacrificed greatly in childhood, we may be able to tolerate great suffering at the hands of our patients, perhaps even masochistically enjoy it, yet not be helping anyone. Also, we may identify with a patient and be able to sacrifice more because of it, experiencing a degree of vicarious affirmation and transformation. I realize that only adequate personal analysis and a relatively high degree of self-awareness can inform these assessments, but they are worthy of aspiration nonetheless.

Over time, I think the inevitable resentment of suffering too much surfaces, and this is when we become martyrs and no one benefits. But the patient may have come to expect the indulgences of the therapist and fear abandonment and loss of connection if these indulgences are withdrawn. This is when things can get really messy. The longer a bad practice continues in a treatment, the more difficult it is to put an end to it. I am convinced generally that when a therapist presents a case where the patient was abusive over time, little therapy was actually taking place. But more recently, I have wondered whether my position might be too idiosyncratic, and that some therapists might gladly suffer even the most difficult, abusive patient.

While speaking at a conference in Poland a few years ago, I listened intently to a presentation by fellow panelist and respected psychoanalyst, Mary Hepworth (nee Target). Dr. Hepworth presented a case that she has talked about many times. She has alternately given this patient the pseudonym of both "Rosa" and "Jenny"; I will use the name "Jenny" in referencing her.

Hepworth began her presentation with the outcome of the treatment, which was impressively positive and highly transformative. She made it clear from the outset that she was the therapist of last resort. Jenny's history included several failed treatments over many years. In a paper about this treatment (Target, 2016), she states,

> Jenny had developed borderline and paranoid personality disorders, and major depression, in adolescence. Jenny had had two periods of psychotherapy, some weeks at 16 with an experienced child psychotherapist who had found her impossible to contain in private practice, and for three years following her hospital

admission. During the latter therapy, Jenny had gradually become reclusive and paranoid, neglecting and harming herself; weeks could pass without her seeing anyone she knew, and she binged, bruised herself and pulled much of her hair out; when we met she was still obese and disfigured. (p. 204)

Hepworth reports seeing her four times per week, then says,

We continued for three further years and she developed a social circle, undertook a creative profession training, and got into her first romantic and sexual relationship, which has worked quite well and been sustained for some years since the end of therapy. (p. 205)

These were impressive results by anyone's standards. I was curious how Hepworth and Jenny had made this type of progress and also curious as to why Hepworth presented the outcome prior to presenting the treatment details. I soon learned why. She began to describe what seemed like a torturous experience. Jenny was volatile, to say the least.

Jenny regularly threw things around in her office and, one day while in the throes of a rage, broke an expensive historic window in Hepworth's office. She verbally assaulted and insulted Hepworth on a regular basis and screamed and yelled with abandon. Hepworth said Jenny refused to leave the session until she was ready and demanded to know things like whether or not Hepworth was married or had children. The soul of patience, Dr. Hepworth quietly tolerated these behaviors, saying in her description of facilitating Jenny's affect regulation,

She swore and threw things when thwarted. I needed to "rewind" to when she had broken away from our focus on something in her mind. The aim was not to *interpret* her excruciating loneliness, envy and so on, but to name them and have Jenny add them to her implicit map of emotional states. (p. 207)

As Dr. Hepworth finished her presentation of this difficult case, the Polish audience was in awe, as was I. But I had many questions.

I directly asked Hepworth about her countertransference. Was she not angry when Jenny behaved so abusively? Did Jenny clean up the messes she made in the office or pay for the broken window? Hepworth said no on both counts. I plainly told her it seemed impossible not to feel angry, and told her I could not have tolerated that behavior or allowed Jenny to refuse to take responsibility for her actions. Many in the audience agreed, but Hepworth very calmly said she simply did not feel angry, either about Jenny's behavior or having to clean up after her. When I asked her privately later in the day if there was something in her background that made this possible, she quickly offered up that her brother had been very angry and disruptive and that she was the quiet "good" child. She envied her brother's freedom to express himself and she loved him. As a result, she receives vicarious gratification form others' angry expressions.

So that explained a great deal. But I was still left with questions. Perhaps Hepworth could tolerate Jenny's aggression because of this element of vicarious gratification. But was it really needed? Did Jenny improve so much because of Hepworth's infinite patience and indulgence or in spite of it? Hepworth's devotion to this patient and commitment to helping her were obvious and inspiring. There is no way to determine whether or not Jenny needed the outsized space Hepworth allowed her to occupy. But it is impossible to argue with the results.

I think this case illustrates much of what I have been talking about thus far in this book. Hepworth and Jenny were a match for numerous reasons, including Hepworth's early experience. In her write-up of this patient, she confirms this when she says,

> The point is not that I had something in common with her, but that something true of me was unconsciously mixed into my recognition of her painful feelings. A trickle of personal reality gets through to the patient, as we focus on them, and it adds contrast to their emotional world. (p. 211)

I also believe that Hepworth's acceptance of Jenny's aggression and envy was made possible, in part, by Jenny's comparable devotion to *her*. I think it is not humanly possible to maintain a positive transference and consistent emotional engagement with someone who is only, or even mostly, aggressive and rejecting. Jenny was capable of engaging her analyst—something I think is vital for a successful treatment.

Also, Hepworth may have been the perfect therapist for Jenny, at least in part, because she was someone with whom she shared certain experiences and was someone Jenny could love. Hepworth describes their mutual recognition and attachment this way:

> Jenny was extremely interested in me, much more for years than she was in herself, and she spoke about this a lot. She did not actually need answers to her many, intrusive factual questions but she did need to know what to expect from me and whether I disliked being with her. I think she had some implicit awareness, listening to me listening to her envious, lonely and humiliated feelings, that she happened to be with someone who had known her own waves of shame and self-attack. (pp. 210–211)

I admire Hepworth's willingness to be transparent about her own early experience and how it contributed positively to her relationship with Jenny and to the treatment outcome. I think she illustrates what I described in Chapter 1 regarding the helpfulness of referencing our own early experience when presenting cases, noting that it can be done without excessive self-revelation. This chapter focuses on how both sacrifice and gratification are essential elements in treatment, and I wanted to use this case because it so boldly illustrates both.

I think it is important to address how our early experiences pre-determine to some extent who we can treat and who we cannot. I could not have tolerated the extent of abuse that Jenny heaped on Dr. Hepworth, even if I believed it was necessary for her to make progress. I simply do not have any need to have that experience and could not have avoided being angry and defensive. Therefore, I would have added myself to the list of people who dismissed her and found her untreatable.

My success with patients and my credentials essentially become meaningless when I am faced with a patient I cannot relate to. Regarding my own fluctuating tolerance with difficult patients, in the first half of my career I successfully treated a number of difficult patients, bearing their insults and complaints with relative equanimity. But as I matured and became aware that submitting to this type of behavior rarely produced good results, I became less tolerant of being treated this way. I like to think that becoming aware of my own excessive guilt and sense of responsibility for others also contributed to me not seeing any value in tolerating abuse and helped me to set better limits with abusive patients. My own vulnerability, of course, also determined my tolerance. For example, shortly after my father died after a long bout with dementia, a psychiatrist I worked with asked if I would accept a patient she thought I was uniquely qualified to treat.

The wife of a prominent young physician, she received extra attention and assistance in finding the right therapist. Everyone involved in this case was delighted that I agreed to meet with her, in spite of her history of being difficult. At the appointed hour, I walked into the waiting room and introduced myself. She immediately gave me a critical once-over and reluctantly shook my hand. As we entered my office, she looked around and said, "Nice office. No wonder you charge so much." Having written about the ideal of a certain mutual courting at the onset of treatment (Maroda, 1999), I didn't think her sarcasm was a good sign. I moved on, of course, and asked her to tell me what she was looking for in treatment. She proceeded to deride the profession in general and say that her previous therapists were idiots. She hoped I was better. She hated her life. She was terribly depressed and no one could help. She added that since I wasn't a real doctor—only a PhD, unlike her husband who was a rising star and an MD—she doubted I would be of much help either. I asked her to tell me more about her reservations about being in treatment and her thoughts about what it meant for me to be a PhD rather than an MD. This conversation went nowhere and was followed by a few more insulting remarks.

I tried to tell myself that I should overcome my distaste for this woman, who clearly was suffering and ambivalent about making herself even the tiniest bit vulnerable. But the more she glared at me, the more I disliked her. Finally, after 45 minutes of stilted conversation, I moved to the topic of whether we should work together. She seemed quite taken aback. She assumed I was going to treat her. I asked how she felt about seeing me, and she said she didn't much care for me, but I was supposedly the best, so she figured there wasn't much choice.

I can't think of a time, before or since, when a prospective patient has been so sullen, cold, and even nasty. I just kept thinking to myself, "I do not like this woman and after losing my father, I just do not need this." I tactfully informed her that I didn't think we were a good match and discussed a referral elsewhere. I knew my referral source was going to be quite displeased with this outcome. But I also knew I absolutely could not do a good job with that patient at that point in my life. Retrospectively, I wonder how much she unconsciously knew about my emotional state when she met me. Did she sense I was recovering from some significant loss? Did she need someone who could handle her insults and saw that I bristled at them instead? As a follow-up, I heard from the referring psychiatrist that this patient had accepted my referral to another therapist and was doing well with her.

As I mentioned earlier, that is why I encourage supervisees to ask themselves at the outset whether or not they can be effectively emotionally engaged with a prospective patient. Luchner et al. (2008) illustrate my point about how our ideal of selflessness impacts our self-esteem and colors our clinical choices.

> The therapist may also feel that his or her ability to be selfless is proof that he or she is capable and that without his or her ability to make specific concessions for clients he or she would be negligent and deficient in his or her role as a psychotherapist. (p. 11)

When I presented this concept of the match to a group of seasoned clinicians, they almost all felt obligated to at least attempt to treat anyone who was referred to them. The chorus from the audience was, "If I don't treat this difficult patient, who will?" I responded by saying that's like saying "you have to date anyone who asks you out—otherwise they might end up alone"—which got a laugh, but didn't necessarily change their attitudes. Bacal and Thomson (1996) make the interesting point that some therapists actually thrive on conflict with their patients, in spite of being the minority. And they bring home my point that there is someone for everyone—including the most aggressive patients.

> We recognize that not all analysts find adversarial situation difficult or disaffirming. In fact, some analyst feel mirrored or stimulated by the cut and thrust of an aversive encounter, as do some patients. The different personalities and theoretical approached of analysts indicate great variation in their selfobject needs and expectations. The number of permutations and combinations in mutual selfobject needs, and frustration of such needs, in the psychoanalytic situation must be infinite. (p. 33)

I think this quote helps illustrate the complexity and diversity inherent in the analytic dyad. The fact that we have shared early experiences and motivations for becoming therapists does not negate our unique qualities. If we could only reach the point where we can think about our needs and limitations in concert with our strengths, begin to think more deeply how this potentially works or doesn't work with each new patient, I think analytic theory and practice could be significantly advanced. With our own vulnerabilities and needs in mind, we are in a position to make better choices about who we treat and how we intervene. As Wilson (2003) observes,

> The issue is not simply what kinds of experiences the analyst seeks to re-create or redress by doing analytic work. The issue is how these desired experiences interact with the analyst's conception of the patient's problems, as well as with the patient's own goals and desires for treatment. As I noted earlier, the analytic couple's idiosyncratically evolving interaction of desires, subtly negotiated over time determines the tone and quality of clinical process and outcome. (p. 80)

Gratification and benefit[1]

Perhaps the most obvious, yet unstated, need we have as therapists is a need for intimacy. In a group conversation following an analytic meeting decades ago, the eight or ten of us sitting around waiting to leave for the airport happened upon a discussion of what we get out of being therapists. The one thing that stood out from that conversation was how we laughingly agreed that we are all "intimacy junkies."

We have a low tolerance for small talk, feeling an indescribable sense of unease when we cannot go deeper. The world of feeling is where we want to reside—it is where we feel most comfortable. Farber et al. (2005), in their paper on why therapists choose their vocation, said "Farber and Heifetz (1981) suggested that the combination of helping clients and feeling close to them—what they termed 'intimate involvement'—serves as a particularly strong reward" (p. 107). This may be innate and related to our heightened empathic skills, may be a response to the distress in our families of origin, or both. Whatever its origins, the need for emotional intimacy appears to be one the most compelling motivations for the work we do.

Perhaps no topic is more controversial than that of the analyst's needs being met in the course of treating the patient. Prior emphasis has been placed on satisfaction derived from the patient's progress, with frequent warnings regarding the analyst's inappropriate pursuit of her narcissistic needs. I readily acknowledge that all manner of inappropriate gratification does exist and harms both analyst and patient. Yet, the major thesis presented here states that mutuality is a driving principle in all human relationships. If this is true, then anything that is essentially harmful to the patient is also harmful to the analyst. But it also means that if the analytic relationship facilitates self-discovery and therapeutic transformation of the patient, while providing a sustaining level of affirmation, safety, and well-being, similar benefits will occur for the analyst.

Legitimate gratification of the analyst's needs is both difficult to define and controversial. That we are gratified in our work is self-evident and has been discussed in numerous ways. When it comes to legitimate gratification, however, the favored emphasis has been on seeing the patient change or on vicarious gratification derived from the patient working through conflicts and expressing intense feeling. The notion of any ongoing gratification for the analyst as an inherent part of a successful treatment, especially the notion that the patient helps the analyst to change, or provides emotional or intellectual sustenance for the analyst, remains foreign. Although I use the term gratification throughout, I am referring not merely to immediate pleasure, relief, or satisfaction. *I am referring primarily to a deeper experience of shared deep emotion, personal growth, fulfillment, and transformation for the analyst as a requisite consequence of the analytic process.*

For all the conversations about the inevitability of the analyst's participation as a human being, we are still preoccupied with fears of losing control, of being too needy, or being narcissistic and self-indulgent. What seems odd to me is that for all the emphasis on mutuality in current theory, we do not seriously contemplate that it might be necessary for the analyst to get better if the patient is to get better. And we seem to live in fear of our neediness spilling out uncontrollably and ruining the treatment. Does the extent of this fear reflect on just how needy we really are and how much we deny it? If so, perhaps a more realistic assessment of our own mental health and motivations for doing treatment (Brenner, 1985; Maroda, 1991; Searles, 1979; Sussman, 1992, 1995) must precede any serious consideration of legitimate gratification.

Ferenczi (1932) openly discussed the analyst's need for the patient. But his discussion of the topic has received little attention, even with the resurgence of interest in his work and the expunging of his blackened reputation in the analytic community (Aron & Harris, 1993). It seems that talking about having our needs met by our patients makes us queasy. Bacal and Thomson (1998) represent two of the few voices that have taken up the notion of the analyst's gratification and need for emotional support within the treatment. They point out that traditionally we were not supposed to need our patients' responsiveness, and, out of our shame for having our needs met, we disavow that we even receive anything substantial from them.

> We believe that analysts regularly expect patients to respond in a number of ways that are, in fact, self-sustaining or self-enhancing. And our patients ongoingly meet a number of psychological needs that enable us to go on treating them. For the most part, we are unaware that this is happening ... The analyst's experience of the patient's unresponsiveness is in essence no different from the patient's experience of the analyst's unresponsiveness. When the patient experiences this, we call it a disruption. When the analyst has this experience, we call it countertransference. (pp. 253–254)

Wolf (1998), writing in the same volume edited by Bacal, speaks of the inevitability, not only of the analyst serving as the patient's selfobject but also of the patient serving as the analyst's self-object.

Although these authors do not use the term "mutuality," clearly this is what we are discussing.

Aron (1996) notes that the literature on therapist gratification is sparse, conflict-filled, and remains outside the mainstream. He cites specific analysts from Ferenczi to Winnicott, Jung, Searles, Fromm, Thompson, Tauber, Singer, Levenson, Wolstein, and Bacal, all of whom make some mention of the therapeutic benefit for the analyst. I would add Bellak and Faithorn (1981) to that list, as well as the aforementioned references to the work of Wolf. And I am sure there are others. The observation that the patient cures, heals, gratifies, and soothes the analyst, as well as frustrating and upsetting her, is certainly not a new one. But it appears that the analyst's gratification is something we are more comfortable with in theory than in practice. Even Aron does not get into specifics when he speaks of the inevitability of emotional gratification for the analyst. And Mitchell (1997) says,

> not only is psychoanalysis a powerful, transformative experience for the patient, it also provides an extraordinary experience for the analyst. It is only in recent years, with the increasing openness in writing about countertransference, that it has been possible to acknowledge how absorbing, personally touching, and potentially transformative the practice of psychoanalysis can often be for the analyst. (p. 35)

Mitchell argues for a mutually transformative process but does not go so far as to confirm my view that some degree of transformation for the analyst *necessarily occurs* in a successful treatment.

Szasz (1956) wrote the only article that directly speaks, at least theoretically, to the inevitability of mutual and deep gratification in the analytic relationship. He speaks to why we tend to deny our knowledge of mutual gratification.

> The fact remains ... that while this "knowledge" about the analyst's gratifications "exists," it is at best latent and is unacknowledged officially. It seems to me fair to assert, first, that little emphasis is placed in our theory in general, and in discussions of techniques in particular, on this aspect of the analytic situation;

and secondly, that on the contrary, we frequently encounter authors dwelling at great length on the emotional hardships to which the analyst is subjected by the nature of his work. Is it not possible that from the point of view of psychological science this socially condoned position of the analyst is not altogether honest? (pp. 210–211)

As usual, Szasz was ahead of his time in his insinuation that the analyst is not fessing up to the full realities of her personal involvement in the analytic relationship. He talks about the quandary we face when attempting to answer the question, "Who needs whom, and how much?" (p. 212). While he considers this question inherently unanswerable, he warns us against the passive acceptance of the patient as the primary beneficiary of the analytic process.

Szasz likens the analyst–patient relationship to the parent–child, clergy–worshipper, leader–follower, and other "fundamental paired systems" that rely on the attribution of neediness to one person in the pair providing power and prestige to the other. He labels the belief that one member receives gratification while the other is self-sacrificing as "the great over-simplification." He cautions us that

> there is no safeguard against the hazard of the patient re-experiencing in his relationship with the analyst a human interaction significantly similar to that between a child and a masochistic, "self-sacrificing" parent. The burdens and inhibitions which such a relationship can place on the developing child's ego are familiar enough to us and do not require further comment. (p. 221)

I agree with Szasz that the answer to the question, "Who needs whom, and how much?" is unanswerable even in the general sense, let alone with regard to each unique analytic pair. But, again, do we not need to strive for the highest levels of self-awareness, even when it comes to our own neediness? We know our knowledge will always be imperfect. We also know that the price for denial can be substantial. I think Szasz is right when he says that the long-suffering analyst poses as much of a threat to the patient as the long-suffering parent did.

A review of the recent literature produced only one article on the topic of legitimate gratification, "On Gratitude and Gratification"

(Gabbard, 2000). He provides a case example of a patient who made a point of negating Gabbard's influence over him and withholding any expression of appreciation or gratitude, which frustrated Gabbard. Generalizing beyond the scope of his work with this patient, he says,

> Indeed, our contemplation of the patient's gratitude leads us directly into considerations related to the analyst's gratification. The wish for something in return from our patients, and the longing for expressions of gratitude and appreciation, is related to our unconscious motivations for choosing a career as an analyst. In addition to our altruistic intentions, most of us are searching for some form of healing in our work ... We offer understanding, caring and affirmation, but we hope to receive gratitude and appreciation for our efforts. (p. 698)

Obviously, Gabbard is on to something when he says we need something from our patients, but I disagree with his conclusion. I think we often settle for gratitude, seeking it or complaining about not getting it only when our deeper needs for affirmation are not met. Focusing on gratitude is what you do in an interpersonal relationship when you feel someone owes you something. Implicitly, it means that the relationship is tilted out of mutuality. When both people's needs are being met, gratitude, while it may be present, is not at the forefront.

One of the simplest and earliest contributions on gratification comes from Fine (1986).

> Our patients are by and large better educated, in better economic circumstances and, most paradoxical of all, in better mental health that most of the people in our society. Thus, inherently even the everyday work of analysis is gratifying in many ways. (p. 19)

Having some idea about how our needs are being met in the analytic process is invaluable to the work we do. I believe that it is our frustrated needs and lack of overall gratification with individual patients that lead us to improper or untherapeutic attempts at gratification. So my hypothesis states that illegitimate gratification results from thwarted legitimate gratification, which brings up the interesting notion that patients who actively seek sex, late-night phone calls, vacation contact, and other questionable gratifications from the analyst may be settling for these things because they cannot get what they really need.

How many patients settle for extending the session a few extra minutes, or calling the analyst at home, when they feel they have not been heard or adequately responded to? I have always wondered why some therapists get incessant phone calls and demands for special favors from their needy patients, while others get few or none. Whereas this phenomenon may be explained, in part, by the patient's knowledge of what the analyst is or is not willing to do, or what the analyst has or does not have to give, I think it may also be a function of what the patient is actually getting in the sessions.

The difficulty in pursuing the notion of legitimate gratification harkens back to the aforementioned fears of illegitimate gratification. How can we know when our pleasure and satisfaction occur in tandem with the patient's transformation or at his expense? It is safe to say that any form of gratification that violates the boundaries of the professional relationship cannot be considered legitimate and in the best interest of either participant. It is easy to name some clearly defined instances of therapist abuse, such as repeatedly telling one's personal problems to patients, making any business deals or taking insider stock tips from patients, having extra-analytic contact with patients, and having intimate physical contact with them.

We may try to "get something" from the patient through therapist-initiated phone calls or appointments, therapist-initiated emphasis on the positive transference (including the erotic or loving transference), or focusing on any topic within a session that may capture the therapist's interest but not be really important to the patient. Or we may fail to support the patient's attempts to cut down on sessions or set a termination date, be chronically late for sessions, frequently reschedule sessions, or take non-emergency phone calls during sessions. If these behaviors are anomalies (and not due to some personal crisis in the analyst's life), I would ask how and why the analyst feels personally or professionally frustrated in relation to this particular patient at this time. If these behaviors occur across patients, I would suggest that this analyst has unresolved issues that motivate her to seek power and personal convenience at her patients' expense.

Crastnopol (1999) and Aron (2000) have also written about potential intrusions into the treatment through the analyst writing about patients. These analysts note that writing about patients can be a form of legitimate gratification as well, just as suggesting an extra session may be in the patient's best interest during some difficult time. I always get my patient's consent to write about them, even in the most disguised form, and encourage a period of thoughtfulness about this. Since I treat a number of therapists, I have found that their initial reaction is to say "yes," followed by ambivalence. When I pursue this, most of them have let me know they prefer not to be discussed, even if they are given the material to review before I use it. This necessarily removes quite a bit of interesting case material I would have liked to use. But respecting their desire for privacy and their fears of becoming responsible for my needs are well worth the sacrifice. Other patients are fine with being included, or even a bit tickled by it, and I do write about them. Regardless of a yes or no answer, I encourage paying attention to dreams and being candid with me following a request to be written about.

Defining legitimate gratification within the parameters of the relationship presents even greater difficulties. The gray area that Gabbard calls "boundary crossings"—temporary alterations in the professional stance, such as hugging the patient, that may be therapeutic—can be the most difficult to assess. We can legitimize emotional gratification for the analyst while still maintaining the old standard that the analyst's behavior should be responsive to the patient's need. What we speak less of is that even if the patient initiates the hug, it must be a positive experience for the analyst as well. Otherwise the analyst is avoiding one pitfall—the narcissistic injury suffered by the patient when a hug is refused (McLaughlin, 1995)—while falling prey to another: the tension and implicit rejection of the contact communicated by the analyst's discomfort. In order for the encounter to be therapeutic, both parties must feel comfortable. And sometimes we have to make a mistake before we know what works, and what does not, with a particular patient, or to discover what we ourselves are comfortable doing or not doing. Lastly, we have to come to terms with the possibility that a patient may genuinely need something that we simply cannot give.

When I was presenting at a conference some years ago, a therapist in the audience asked me about a patient she was treating who recently began hugging her hard at the end of each session. The therapist perceived this patient as easily wounded, so she did not bring the hugs up for discussion to avoid humiliating her. The therapist assumed the hugs were temporary and that the patient would broach the topic at some point in the treatment. She stated it had now been two months, and there was no end in sight. What did I think?

I advised her on two fronts. First, what happened two months ago? The question of "why now?" is rarely out of my immediate consciousness. Second, if the goal is emotional honesty, and if the therapist believes in mutuality, then how can she continue to accept the hugs? Isn't her increasing discomfort the proverbial elephant in the room? I encouraged her to gently tell the patient at the start of the next session that she was wondering about the hugs and what she might be needing from the therapist and not getting. I also encouraged her to engage the patient as a consultant on her own case, asking what she thought about what might have happened between them two months ago that made the patient feel the need for this fervent physical contact. (For the record, the therapist did reveal a personal problem of her own that led to her being less emotionally available at that time.)

I think there are two principles that can guide the analyst in making good decisions. The first guiding principle is the aforementioned mutuality. I believe that it is virtually impossible to do or say things over time that are bad for the patient but good for the analyst. Analysts who gratify themselves at their patients' expense invariably feel guilt and shame and know that things are not as they should be. Past permissions to write off the patient's complaints or symptoms as transference only facilitate the analyst's denial that something is awry. Sadly, the analyst may not become aware of what she is doing until disaster strikes. Serious boundary violations carry the threat of ethical or criminal charges, painful lawsuits, and public humiliation for the analyst.

I want to reemphasize the aspect of "over time" with respect to what is mutually beneficial. Certainly, all of us do satisfy some immediate need or desire at the other person's expense in any relationship—and sometimes for good reason in terms of our own survival. And we are equally familiar with the frequency of competing needs in any relationship. Stand-offs inevitably occur when both parties are needy and in an incompatible direction. I approach the topic of mutually beneficial, growth-producing therapeutic relationships with the knowledge that this must be a relative concept. The therapeutic relationship cannot transcend the limitations of all human relationships, which necessarily include periods of insensitivity, neglect, power-seeking, and even some degree of exploitation. The point is not to create an unattainable ideal, but rather to point out that a certain amount of therapist gratification, both superficial and deep, necessarily occurs in tandem with the patient's improvement.

An ongoing obstacle to the analyst trusting her feelings of unease, guilt, or shame over what is happening in the therapeutic relationship is the irrational guilt and shame discussed by Bacal and Thomson. If we feel guilt and shame about having any of our needs met, if we feel guilt and shame over enjoying the patient and laughing at his jokes or looking forward to seeing him, if we feel guilt and shame over discovering a part of ourselves that we have never really known before, then guilt and shame no longer serve as reliable signals that something is awry in the relationship. Many therapists still feel guilt and shame over having intense feelings about a patient, particularly sexual ones, or over having felt better as a result of being with the patient. I believe that this has to change.

Therapists who act out destructively with their patients have often been unbearably frustrated in the relationship for some time and cannot find their way out. They settle for what they can get, or they allow an abusive patient to get away with behaving badly, not paying the fee, or harassing the analyst during his private time outside the sessions. If they cannot feel competent, they may settle for feeling desired.

Consultations may fail to help the situation because they rarely focus on the true needs of both analyst and patient. From my experience, consultants usually provide well-intentioned support for their colleagues' insights and feelings. Historically, we have not asked, "What does the analyst need that he or she is not getting?" and can this situation be changed in a way that is therapeutic for the patient? If not, how can the therapist attend to her emotional needs outside the analytic relationship so that she is in a better position to facilitate the treatment?

Therapy relationships, like all relationships, tend to be mutually gratifying or mutually frustrating, either in the general sense or at any point in time. Whether the difficulty is ongoing, intermittent, or rare, I think it is vital that the analyst be able to say to herself, without guilt or shame, how am I emotionally frustrated in this relationship? How is this patient not functioning as a self object for me? And how am I failing to function as a good-enough self-object for the patient? Are either of us denying our need or feelings for each other? Does this patient have a history of not giving over to others? Do I have a history of not making myself vulnerable? How is each of us contributing to our mutually frustrated state and what needs to happen to create or restore our mutual self-object status?

This leads us to the second principle that can help us to decide whether we are indulging ourselves or responding to the patient. Has the patient taken the initiative or has the analyst? Everything from self-disclosure to physical contact to advice-giving has been shown to be therapeutic primarily when the patient rather than the analyst initiates it. Granted, when we are talking about projective identification or enactment, the notion of who is initiating can be very difficult to ascertain. I think the best we can do is simply ask ourselves, "Am I doing this in response to the patient or is my behavior born out of my own curiosity, opinions, neediness, or defensiveness?" Again, knowing that we have unconscious motivations that preclude us from certainty should not deter us from pursuing self-awareness.

Conclusion

We have long recognized the role of self-sacrifice as we carry out our task of doing analytic treatment. But we have been far less forthcoming when it comes to the necessity of meeting certain of our own needs in the process of helping our patients. With the resurgence of discussions about surrender and self-sacrifice, I think it important not to endorse masochism. It is equally important to personally assess our own needs for doing treatment and understand how those are met, both in the general sense and with each individual patient. Those needs necessarily change in accordance with our age, experience, and life situations, which demands ongoing self-awareness. The goal proposed here is to achieve a healthy balance between self-sacrifice and gratification, knowing that this is not only in our best interest but also in our patients'. In the next chapter, I will address the specific needs that are frequently met by doing psychotherapy and psychoanalysis, as well as the role of both our shared and unique vulnerabilities.

Note

1 Much of what follows in this chapter was previously published as Maroda (2005).

References

Akhtar, S., & Varma, A. (2012). Sacrifice: Psychodynamic, cultural and clinical aspects. *The American Journal of Psychoanalysis, 72*, 95–117.

Alford, C. F. (2000). Levinas and Winnicott: Motherhood and responsibility. *American Imago, 57*, 235–259.

Aron, L. (2000). Ethical considerations in the writing of psychoanalytic case histories. *Psychoanalytic Dialogues, 10*, 231–245.

Aron, L. (1996). *A meeting of minds.* Hillsdale, NJ: The Analytic Press.

Aron, L., & Harris, A. (Eds.) (1993). *The legacy of Sandor Ferenczi.* Hillsdale, NJ: The Analytic Press.

Bacal, H. A., & Thomson, P. G. (1996). The psychoanalyst's selfobject needs and the effect of their frustration on the treatment: A new view of countertransference. *Progress in Self Psychology, 12*, 17–35.

Bacal, H. A., & Thomson, P. G. (1998). Optimal responsiveness and the therapist's reaction to the patient's unresponsiveness. In H. Bacal (Ed.), *Optimal responsiveness: How therapists heal their patients* (pp. 249–270). Northvale, NJ: Aronson.

Bellak, L., & Faithorn, P. (1981). *Crises and special problems in psychoanalysis and psychotherapy.* New York: Brunner/Mazel.

Blau, P. M. (1964). *Exchange and power in social life.* New York: Wiley.

Brenner, C. (1985). Countertransference as a compromise formation. *Psychoanalytic Quarterly, 54*, 155–163.

Celenza, A. (2007). *Sexual boundary violations: Therapeutic, supervisory, and academic contexts.* New York: Aronson.

Coen, S. J. (2000). The wish to regress in patient and analyst. *Journal of the American Psychoanalytic Association, 48*, 785–810.

Crastnopol, M. (1999). The analyst's professional self as a "third" influence on the dyad: When the analyst writes about the treatment. *Psychoanalytic Dialogues, 9*, 445–470.

Downey, G., Freitas, A. L., Michaelis, B., & Khouri, H. (1998). The self-fulfilling prophecy in close relationships: Rejection sensitivity and rejection by romantic partners. *Journal of Personality and Social Psychology*, *75*(2), 545–560.

Farber, B. A., & Heifetz, L. J. (1981). The satisfactions and stresses of psychotherapeutic work: A factor analytic study. *Professional Psychology*, *12*(5), 621–630.

Farber, B. A., Manevich, J., Metzer, J., & Saypol, E. (2005). Choosing psychotherapy as a career: Why did we cross that road? *Journal of Clinical Psychology*, *61*, 1009–1031.

Ferenczi, S. (1988, 1932). *The clinical diary of Sándor Ferenczi* (J. Dupont, Ed.; M. Balint & N. Z. Jackson, Trans.). Cambridge, MA: Harvard University Press.

Fine, R. (1986). Countertransference and the pleasures of being an analyst. *Current Issues in Psychoanalytic Practice*, *2*, 3–19.

Gabbard, G. (1995). The early history of boundary violations in psychoanalysis. *Journal of the American Psychoanalytic Association*, *43*, 1115–1136.

Gabbard, G. (2000). On gratitude and gratification. *Journal of the American Psychoanalytic Association*, *48*, 697–716.

Ghent, M. (1990). Masochism, submission, surrender—Masochism as a subversion of surrender. *Contemporary Psychoanalysis*, *26*, 108–136.

Impett, E. A., Gable, S. L., & Peplau, L. A. (2005). Giving up and giving in: The costs and benefits of daily sacrifice in intimate relationships. *Journal of Personality and Social Psychology*, *89*, 327–344.

Kravis, N. (2013). The analyst's hatred of analysis. *Psychoanalytic Quarterly*, *82*, 89–114.

Lerner, M. J., Miller, D. T., & Holmes, J. G. (1976). Deserving vs justice: A contemporary dilemma. In L. Berkowitz & E. Walster (Eds.), *Advances in experimental social psychology* (Vol. 9, pp. 169–193). New York: Academic Press.

Levinas, E. (1986). Dialogues with Emmanuel Levinas. In R. Cohen (Ed.), *Face to face with Levinas* (pp. 13–34). Albany: State University of New York Press.

Luchner, A. F., Mirsalimi, H., Moser, C. J., & Jones, R. A. (2008). Maintaining boundaries in psychotherapy: Covert narcissistic personality characteristics and psychotherapists. *Psychotherapy: Theory, Research, Practice, Training*, *45*(1), 1–14.

Maroda, K. (1991). *The power of countertransference*. Chichester, UK: Wiley.

Maroda, K. (1999). *Seduction, surrender, and transformation: Emotional engagement in the analytic process*. Hillsdale, NJ: The Analytic Press.

Maroda, K. (2005). Legitimate gratification of the analyst's needs. *Contemporary Psychoanalysis*, *41*, 371–388.

McLaughlin, J. (1995). Touching limits in the analytic dyad. *Psychoanalytic Quarterly, 64,* 433–465.

Mitchell, S. (1997). *Influence and autonomy in psychoanalysis.* Hillsdale, NJ: The Analytic Press.

Orange, D. M. (1995). *Emotional understanding: Studies in psychoanalytic epistemology.* New York: Guilford Press.

Orange, D. M. (2016a). *Nourishing the inner life of clinicians and humanitarians: The ethical turn in psychoanalysis.* London: Routledge.

Orange, D. M. (2016b). Is ethics masochism? On infinite ethical responsibility and finite human capacity. In D. M. Goodman & E. R. Severson (Eds.), *The ethical turn* (pp. 57–74). London: Routledge.

Pinsky, E. (2011). The Olympian delusion. *Journal of the American Psychoanalytic Association, 59,* 351–375.

Righetti, F., & Impett, E. (2017). Sacrifice in close relationships: Motives, emotions, and relationship outcomes. *Social and Personality Psychology Compass.* DOI: https://doi.org/10.1111/spc3.12342.

Rosenblatt, P. (2009). Providing therapy can be therapeutic for a therapist. *American Journal of Psychotherapy, 63,* 169–181.

Searles, H. (1979). *Countertransference and related subjects.* New York: International Universities Press.

Shapiro, Y., & Gabbard, G. O. (1994). A reconsideration of altruism from an evolutionary and psychodynamic perspective. *Ethics & Behavior, 4*(1), 23–42.

Shulman, M. (2016). "Unavoidable satisfactions": The analyst's pleasure. *Journal of the American Psychoanalytic Association, 64,* 697–727.

Sussman, M. (1992). *A curious calling.* New York: Aronson.

Sussman, M. (1995). *A perilous calling: The hazards of psychotherapy practice.* New York: Wiley.

Szasz, T. (1956). On the experience of the analyst in the psychoanalytic situation. *Journal of the American Psychoanalytic Association, 4,* 197–223.

Target, M. (2016). Mentalization within intensive analysis with a borderline patient. *British Journal of Psychotherapy, 32,* 202–214.

Van Lang, P. A. M., Drigotas, S. M., Rusbult, C. E., Arriage, X. B., Witcher, B. S., & Cox, C. L. (1997). Willingness to sacrifice in close relationships. *Journal of Personality and Social Psychology, 72,* 1373–1395.

Wilson, M. (2003). The analyst's desire and the problem of narcissistic resistances. *Journal of the American Psychoanalytic Association, 51,* 71–99.

Wolf, E. (1998). Optimal responsiveness and disruption-restorations. In H. Bacal (Ed.), *Optimal responsiveness: How therapists heal their patients* (pp. 237–248). Northvale, NJ: Aronson.

Chapter 3

The analyst's narcissistic vulnerability

To be an effective analyst or therapist requires one to be vulnerable. Being hurt, disappointed, discouraged, and even humiliated are just as inevitable as our shared joy and pathos (Chused, 2012). There has been much discussion regarding whether or not analysts are more narcissistically vulnerable than other professionals. For many years, I agreed with Luchner et al. (2008), Wilson (2003), Seligson (1992), Sussman (1992), Finell (1985), and others who suggested that we might be. However, after 35 years of treating people from every walk of life, I have concluded that therapists do not seem to be more narcissistically organized than others.

Nevertheless, our narcissistic needs can present a significant obstacle to effective treatment. Our disavowal of narcissistic needs, in particular, creates an obvious barrier to identifying when and how they are obstructing the treatment process. Finell (1985) wrote persuasively about the analyst's narcissistic needs more than three decades ago, emphasizing personal analysis as the only antidote to pervasive, and largely unconscious processes present in the narcissistic defenses of "splitting, denial, and projection" (p. 433).

If Finell is correct in assuming that the most narcissistic gratifications on the analyst's part will necessarily be out of awareness, is there any hope for an optimal degree of self-awareness? What should analysts look for as signs of healthy gratification versus the analyst gratifying himself at his patient's expense? What attitudes on the analyst's part suggest a healthy perspective on himself and his work, and what attitudes represent a denial of needs and feelings that may be egodystonic? And how do these attitudes spill over into the analytic community as a whole? In line with the theme of this book, what are the origins of the analyst's vulnerability and narcissistic needs? And to what extents do analysts display healthy versus unhealthy narcissism?

This chapter is devoted to examining our inevitable narcissistic vulnerabilities as human beings. The objective here is to remove the stigma of vulnerability and open up discussion and greater self-reflection on the analyst's part. Discarding the accusation of pathological narcissism as rampant in the analytic community and replacing it with ideas about how our early experiences might contribute to certain types of vulnerability will hopefully open new areas for self-examination.

Uses and misuses of the term *narcissism*

As many authors have noted (e.g., Pulver, 1970), the terms *narcissism* and *narcissistic* have become overburdened in the last four decades. Even within the profession, it has become easy to use the term *narcissistic* as a pejorative label (Hirsch, 2011, 2014) rather than one describing a particular area(s) of vulnerability.

Colloquial definitions of narcissism are all too familiar. Centered on grandiosity, defensiveness, and a lack of empathy and introspection, I do not believe most therapists fit this description. Nor do simplistic judgments do justice to the complexity of character that allows for the existence of kindness and empathy, while also allowing for bouts of defensive envy, power-seeking, and the need to be special. This chapter will examine the concepts of our narcissistic vulnerability, its roots in childhood experiences, the resulting shame that often interferes with awareness and acceptance of vulnerability, the awareness of healthy narcissism and meeting of our needs, and our need to be affirmed by our patients in an ongoing way.

I have always preferred the concept of *narcissistic vulnerability* and *narcissistic injury*, whether in reference to my patients or to myself and my colleagues. I find these terms incisively descriptive and applicable to virtually everyone. We are vulnerable and we all suffer assaults on our self-esteem. So these terms can be used to aptly describe areas where individuals are prone to blows to their self-esteem and to equally identify when the circumstances under which those blows were felt, without assigning insulting labels. Judith Chused (2012) has written poignantly and straightforwardly about the therapeutic necessity of our narcissistic vulnerability in the sense that I am describing it. She also notes the dearth of discussion on the topic.

> But what has not yet been explored is our own narcissism, our vulnerability, and how to use it and the defensive reactions it stimulates in us, to understand and help our patients. To the extent we are invested in an analysis, we will be narcissistically vulnerable, and we must be so invested for the analysis to be genuinely mutative for the patient. *Difficulties develop not when we are narcissistically injured or elated, but when injury or grandiosity are not recognized or tolerated.* (p. 900, emphasis added)

The analytic ideal has historically downplayed the analyst's vulnerability to being hurt and shamed, along with the inevitable defensive responses that result. Acknowledging that we can be, and are, hurt or embarrassed on a regular basis, and that feeling defensive is natural and human, can relieve the analyst of the need to deny these feelings. It can also serve to help us identify our defensiveness in the moment so that we can productively work through it with the patient. The problem is that our analytic ideal is so unrealistic that we are prone to *feeling defensive about being defensive.* Feeling threatened and being defensive become additional unacceptable flaws.

There is little room to navigate once that position takes hold. Again, now that we take the patient's complaints and critique of us quite seriously, rather than writing it off as transference, we are arguably more vulnerable (Eagle, 2007; Gill, 1984; Hirsch, 2008). Sometimes it seems that we have lost track of the fact that the patient comes to us with his or her own history that can be played out with great distortion as well as great clarity. How do we currently manage these two realities: first, that both people in the analytic dyad begin the relationship with long-established ways of seeing and emotionally experiencing the world; and second, that we ideally create something new between us that is transformative? We have been discouraged from looking at the patient's responses to us as distortions, let alone outright fabrications, in the interest of taking the patient seriously and being open to his or her criticisms of us.

It is unacceptable in the analytic world to blame the patient for our responses, which is something we all applaud. But seemingly without a new paradigm that sufficiently addresses either the patient's distortions or our own, how do we navigate the relationship in a way that recognizes both the healthy and unhealthy aspects of our ways of relating? How often do we manage our own negative participation with a new version of "the patient made me do it" by attributing our behaviors to inevitable enactments? (This is the topic of Chapter 5.) Have we gone too far in letting ourselves and our patients off the hook for unhealthy or morally questionable behavior by conscripting it to the realm of unconsciously driven repetition?

The reluctance to diagnose or to categorize our patients' interpersonal and intrapsychic dilemmas, as well as our own, leaves us in a gray zone of unknowing. Since labeling of any kind is often seen as pejorative, where does that leave us in terms of acknowledging negative feelings and intentions, or simple bad behavior? Is the end result that no one is really in charge or morally responsible for their behavior?

Although the literature is replete with case histories of enactment, including referencing the analyst's personal issues, there is little or no discussion of actual therapeutic error, let alone character flaws. I say this with the understanding that we all err every day and that these errors, if admitted, can often turn into therapeutic moments. I encourage young therapists to accept that they will make mistakes every day and to be open to seeing and admitting those mistakes as a natural part of our work. I am more concerned with ongoing errors or blind spots created by the analyst who is defending against narcissistic injury or guilt-producing conflict.

Patients can, and do, call us out on our defensive maneuvers. For example, after a particularly hard day, I met with a patient who is difficult to reach emotionally and often prickly, in spite of her strong attachment to me. The following week, I was going to be away on vacation. She was notably distant and silent for a long time at the start of her session. She was pregnant at the time and said she was uneasy about her gynecologist being out of town to attend a conference, even though her due date was not imminent.

I am amazed at how often over the years I have missed a reference to my upcoming absences or even forgotten to tell a needy patient about said absence until the last minute, even though I am well aware that this is not therapeutic. It tends to happen with patients who are particularly upset by my departures, often implying that I am either derelict in my duty toward them or unconcerned about their pain. There are certain times when my need to be free and not struggle with irrational guilt about leaving needy patients overcomes my best judgment and practice as an analyst. This session was just such an occasion.

As it finally dawned on me that she was talking about my vacation and was upset about it, the session was almost over. We were going to meet again later in the week, but I felt compelled to bring up the neglected topic once it came into my awareness. The source of this need was my internal guilt and embarrassment about not having noticed this elephant in the room earlier in the session.

The patient, who is very intelligent and psychologically minded, said to me, "So you bring this up right at the end of the session when there's no time to address it? I think you did this to make yourself feel better, and you kid yourself that it's good for me, but it isn't." I was astounded at how correct she was and how quickly she registered that I was attempting to redeem myself before the end of the session, with little thought to the impact on her. When I quickly admitted that she was right, without any defensiveness or self-abnegation, she visibly relaxed.

At other times, the situation is not always so clear to me. Sometimes, a patient will accuse me of bad intentions or insensitivity, and I feel myself squirming inside or scrambling intellectually to rationalize my behavior. But just as with the aforementioned patient, I actually find it relieving to note this to myself and admit it if called upon to do so. My patients are also relieved, of course, and sometimes a bit triumphant over catching me in the act. If I don't need to be perfect, then these moments have great potential to be therapeutic and often become playful.

Early career therapists, in particular, often believe that their vulnerabilities are a sign of weakness, deficiency or failure, which inhibits their open discussion of these inevitable treatment events, as well as their ability to handle them internally. Rather than simply referring to it in the abstract, we need clear clinical examples of the analyst's vulnerability, how it effects the treatment, and how it can be managed. Ignoring the issue of our vulnerability increases our defensiveness as we expect more than is possible. On this topic, Kravis (2013) says,

> Insofar as clinical analytic work presents nearly limitless possibilities for narcissistic injury to the analyst, one should expect to encounter the mobilization of the full range of narcissistic defenses among analysts, both individually and collectively as a professional community. (p. 92)

It goes without saying that our training programs could do better in emphasizing what Kravis is saying. Trainees should be taught to accept early in their careers that it is not about whether you are vulnerable; it is about how and when you are, and what you can do to manage it constructively. Vulnerability is the human condition. Our work ego cannot be so rigid that we expect ourselves to transcend human nature.

Just as with all countertransference, each of us has a pattern of responding that we can identify, track, and keep in mind when doing treatment. I have found the literature on group psychotherapy and psychoanalysis to be particularly useful in this regard. Martin Livingston (2003), in discussing the need for the group analyst's vulnerability in the therapeutic process, reminds us that being vulnerable is no small task and inevitably leads to some wounding of the therapist.

> The word *vulnerable* means "susceptible to being wounded," and people who relinquish their usual characterologic defenses open themselves to wounds of many sets, from peripheral encounters with shame and rejection to direct personal attacks and potentially devastating losses. (p. 648)

I cannot think of a time when anyone in my training told me to expect to be vulnerable and to be hurt, let alone how I would learn to manage that pain. Had I understood that I would necessarily be replaying my own childhood endlessly with patients and that I needed to understand how and why I was vulnerable, I believe that knowledge would have served both my patients and myself. Learning to identify my own patterns of countertransferential responding would have been furthered the process significantly.

Early childhood denial of vulnerability

To what extent is our denial of being hurt at the hands of our patients a carryover from our need to deny hurt at the hands of our parents? Did we feel like failures when we could not rouse a depressed parent from a depressive state? Did we feel inadequate when our caregiver responsibilities seemed like too much—when we chafed at bearing them? And did we feel selfish when we wanted our own needs to take precedence? This could partially explain our reluctance to admit that we have needs in the treatment setting that must be addressed in some fashion.

When we are criticized, do we bristle out of hubris or humiliation? Perhaps analysts may appear to be more narcissistic in the true pathological sense of this term because the treatment process necessarily exposes our vulnerabilities and subsequent shame. We are not surgeons wielding scalpels. Our tools are our powers of observation, emotional honesty, empathic attunement, and willingness to confront both our patients and ourselves.

We appear to seek affirmation and affection, even idealization, from our patients. Yet, we also possess a strong desire to understand and empathize with others—unlikely traits for pathological narcissists. Rather than accepting or dismissing the charge of narcissistic pathology, I think we could gain more from a balanced discussion of how we might collectively share a certain type of narcissistic vulnerability.

Exploring this topic, beginning at the start of training, strikes me as a better way to prepare analysts for both our successes and failures, as well as pointing the way for managing our potential hubris or excessive guilt and shame. How might we be vulnerable to certain attacks or simple disappointments in our work?

In the previous chapter, I made note of the physician's wife who was referred to me by my consulting psychiatrist. A number of high-level people in the psychiatric community were involved in finding the right therapist for this woman, which I was well aware of before agreeing to meet with her. Having treated quite a few difficult patients, I was not concerned that she had a history of failed treatments.

However, the reader may recall that she immediately insulted me by ridiculing my "fancy office," saying that I charged too much, particularly since I was only a PhD, not a high-status MD like her husband. I described disliking her almost immediately and choosing not to work with her. When discussing her in the last chapter, I mentioned my current vulnerability due to the recent death of my father.

What I did not describe is how surprised I was that her comments were hurtful to me. Rather than taking them in stride, I felt knocked off my perch. I was not only hurt and angry, I was embarrassed and ashamed of my intense reaction and seeming inability to manage my own strong emotions. I was also thinking about how unhappy my consulting psychiatrist would be, not to mention the referrals I would *not be receiving* in the future, if I turned this patient away. How could I let this happen? I was not a neophyte therapist. I had been analyzed; I was in my early 50s. And I normally took pride in being able to handle insults with the understanding that they were more about the patient's vulnerability than my own.

Yet as I spoke with this patient, my vulnerability began transitioning to defensive anger. I saw her noticing my tensing body and unhappy expression. As I began to ask myself what was going on, it took only a millisecond for the pain of my father's recent death—my first experience with the loss of a loved one—to register in very intense visceral way. That's when I knew that I was not emotionally ready to treat someone whose own issues dictated her need to "take me on."

I want to emphasize here that although my bereavement greatly increased my vulnerability to an aggressive patient, I am not saying that I have not been, or do not continue to be, vulnerable to my patients in a variety of ways. Again, my current life variables—including age, experience, degree of life satisfaction, number of difficult patients in my caseload, to name a few—are always working to determine my unique vulnerability to any given patient in the moment. I am additionally aware that I will always be somewhat vulnerable to any accusation of lack of commitment or caring as an extension of the childhood expectation that I "fix things." I agree with Frommer (2013) regarding our continued focus on the patient's vulnerability to the exclusion of our own.

It is strangely ironic that while analytic work deals essentially with human suffering, limitation, and loss (Kilborne, 2007), the source of this suffering must be that of the patient and never the analyst. As Brody (this issue) notes, "Though we uncover the painful humanity of our patients, we are loath to reveal our own human-ness." (p. 56)

This attitude has prevented us from pursuing greater insights into regarding the types of vulnerability that might arise as part of who we are and the work we do. One could easily argue that the whole concept of being responsible for healing or comforting others, beginning at an early age, constitutes the high probability of periods of frustration and failure.

Little (1951) argued that perhaps as our patients improve we might countertransferentially need to make them "ill" again so that we could both keep them and revisit our need to heal them. No doubt there is some truth to what she says. But what if this cycle of "making patients better, followed by them being sick again" is also the natural rhythm of making progress, going deeper, and moving on to new issues or facets of old issues that need to be addressed? This is not news to any experienced analyst, but once again, is there a discrepancy between what we know intellectually and how we feel during periods when the patient is distant, newly angry, or critical? To what extent does our need to be connected and useful interfere with the patient's needed periods of consolidation and independence? Is our emphasis on attachment and attunement interfering with a sense of agency for both analyst and patient?

Our need to be special

No doubt there is a particular type of narcissism associated with being a therapist related to our inflated importance as childhood soothers and peacekeepers. On this point, a colleague of mine (Brian Smothers, personal communication) told me he felt that in addition to our deep needs for intimacy, we have a need to feel special that also reprises our childhood experiences. As much as we might have felt deprived of the opportunity to simply be children, we were, indeed, found to be essential to maintaining the family through our high level of empathy and emotional sensitivity.

Taking on this Herculean and impossible task, which we could not recognize as such when we were children, generates self-expectations that we carry throughout our lives. Our inability to make good on these unrealistic expectations is the very definition of shame. Thus, when our patients find us wanting and accuse us of incompetence or lack of caring, our defensive shame is easily mobilized.

Pinsky (2011) refers to the analyst's need to share the patient's idealizations of the analyst and the process as the "Olympian delusion."

> That delusion, even if it has no other harmful effects, blocks the patient's necessary *dis*illusion—a gradual process of mourning that includes acceptance of the analyst as a human being with ordinary defects and limitations. Indeed, only an imperfect, striving mortal can *offer* the doubled gifts of attention and abstinence. A god, or a machine, won't do. (p. 367)

As we were called to take on more responsibility, we also came to inhabit a special place in our families of origin. We were needed and turned to in moments of distress. We were, in a sense, the chosen ones. (I have also observed rather intense sibling rivalries in therapist families, including my own. Siblings are understandably resentful of the special status of the budding therapist.) Smothers believes that we are highly motivated to re-create this special status in relation to our patients, thereby affirming both the value of our sacrifice and our unique abilities. I think he is right. In speaking about this with other therapists, they readily accede that being important to their patients is one of the most gratifying aspects of their work.

This explanation seems to account for both our exquisite vulnerability to being found wanting and our excessive pride in the accomplishments of our patients. Coen (2007) has written non-judgmentally about the rather obvious pride and vicarious pleasure we take in identifying with and treating "special" people.

> What analysts find impressive about their patients can include fame, power, strength, intelligence, wealth, prestige, talent, creativity, abilities, attractiveness, sexiness, youth, seniority—whatever may have special appeal to the needs of a given analyst. But an impressive patient has been made so by the analyst's needs. (p. 1169)

I appreciate Coen's insights regarding the variety of qualities we can be attracted to in our patients, depending on our own needs and early experiences. Coen also notes that we can equally be drawn to patients who reflect our own darker inclinations, as we strive to integrate those inclinations with our need to be good people. I think we are not so different from other people in this regard. Again, the point of emphasizing our own conflicts and deficits is not to imply that we are *not* good people, but rather to shed light on the important consequences for reliving our own pasts with the idiosyncratic context of doing treatment.

Our capacity for empathy and genuine concern is clearly embedded in our emotional sensitivity and capacity for intimacy. This necessarily leaves us vulnerable. If we could embrace a reasonable degree of vulnerability as critical to human connection, even though it translates into missteps at times, perhaps we could better prepare ourselves for doing treatment.

This vulnerability on the analyst's part needed to achieve and sustain emotional engagement can be at odds with the idealized persona referenced throughout this volume. If we think of ourselves as magical healers, as the good mothers rather than the bad ones, how do we accept criticism non-defensively—in the best sense of that word? That is, how do we not merely take a deep breath and steel ourselves against feeling the pain of being criticized or devalued, but actually allow these arrows to reach their target regardless of the consequences for our self-esteem? And then how do we manage our own affect when this occurs? When and how do we say "ouch"? Even stickier, how can we allow ourselves to be vulnerable when we perceive the patient as criticizing us in the service of repeating their own experience with being the recipient of rejection, degradation, even humiliation?

If we accept their observations as reasonably accurate, which they often are, does this make us failed healers? How can we bear this failure to fulfill the reparative countertransference, even in the moment? Greenberg (2001), in his discussion of the analyst's participation, notes that in dealing with patients whose transferences require them to keep us at a distance, we may be too prone to finding fault in ourselves, even if we do not acknowledge it: "I believe that many analysts these days are living with the tension of believing that they could revitalize relationships that have been deadened by toxic transferences if only they were braver, more available, or simply more decent" (p. 136). Taken in context with the previous chapters, we might wonder how much of the evolution of analytic theory and practice in the last two decades has influenced our seeming greater tendency to blame ourselves if our patients aren't improving. The classical analyst did not question himself in any public way when presenting a difficult case, although he may well have in private.

Welt and Herron (1990) make an interesting point when they discuss the intricacies of merging with the patient in the healthiest way possible. They note that we frequently interact with our patients on the basis of either acting out our need to sacrifice and rescue them, or on the basis of defending against any notion that we are not doing right by them. The ideal position, of course, is to be neither indulging nor defending against our need to heal them, but rather holding these feelings in awareness so that they might guide our actions. They say, "After all, the ability to merge with the unconscious without either compulsion to do so or compulsion to avoid doing so is a narcissistic function, a healthy narcissistic function" (p. 26).

Healthy narcissism

It appears that conversations centering on the analyst's self-interest are inevitability tied to fears of pathological narcissism on the analyst's part. I think this is unfortunate. I appreciate that one must consider the possibility of the analyst's' pathological narcissism when discussing the analyst's self-interest. What bothers me is the equating of these two events, as if there is no healthy narcissism—no healthy way for the analyst to have his or her needs met. Certainly, we are ethically charged with the responsibility of asking if we are being gratified at the patient's expense. But are we not equally charged with the capacity to recognize mutual empowerment and satisfaction? Wilson (2013), who speaks eloquently about the naturalness of the analyst's desires, says "Our discomfort with our desiring position involves, I believe, the intimate connection between desire and narcissism. Desire, in other words, smacks too much of 'self-interest'" (p. 438).

I think we would benefit from shifting the narrative to include analyst healthy self-interest rather than assuming exploitive self-indulgence. Luchner et al. (2008) cite their research results indicating that narcissism is, in fact, an essential aspect of many of our most positive traits. Noting that narcissism runs on a continuum, they observe, "It is not inherently unhealthy, as narcissistic strivings potentially allow us to both believe in our abilities and ourselves as well as be able to depend on others in times of stress or need (Kohut, 1971, 1984; Wilson, 2013; Wink, 1996; Wolf, 1988)" (p. 1). And again, quoting Chused's (2012) excellent article, "I don't have an official definition, but for me healthy narcissism is having a sense of self that can withstand the blows of failure and rejection, without resorting to grandiosity, paranoia, or projection" (p. 912).

Healthy narcissism is postulated on having sufficiently worked through our childhood need to rescue, thereby utilizing sublimation more than reaction formation. We can also sublimate the need to be special and idealized through effective clinical work that earns the patient's genuine gratitude, respect, and love. In other words, we can actually earn our need to be special through our clinical acumen, as opposed to shoring up a fragile self that needs constant affirmation, whether or not it is deserved.

Greater self-awareness of our needs in general, of course, can help mitigate the need to satisfy them in relation to the patient. In the professional realm, I receive gratification from my writing, presenting, supervising, and mentoring. These other forms of gratification serve to minimize what I need from my patients. The same can be said for my personal relationships. However, there remains in all of us a deeper, more primitive need to be validated by our patients that outside gratifications cannot erase. For all of our conversations about self-care, I think more emphasis early in training on constructive gratification of our narcissistic needs would be more specific and germane to the question of how much we need our patients.

The concept of healthy narcissism and gratification seems highly underrated in our profession. Again, Sussman (1992) pointed out the benefits of the therapist's narcissistic investment some time ago: "The therapist's fulfillment of average expectable narcissistic needs with the treatment setting will not necessarily hinder the therapeutic process, and may actually promote it by simulating the therapist's interest and emotional investment in the patient" (p. 102).

Discussions of the need for personal gratification remain almost nonexistent. This attitude translates into a reluctance to discuss technique, because our needs would become an essential element of that conversation within a two-person paradigm. Again, a review of the literature on the analyst's needs and vulnerabilities is sparse, indeed. In a discussion of the analyst's narcissism and self-disclosure, Kuchuck (2009) says, "Though growing, I suspect that the still relative paucity of literature on this topic may in part be explained by how uncomfortable it makes us feel" (p. 1008). Exactly.

Yet, confronting our own discomfort is ultimately relieving, just as it is for our patients. We achieve a higher level of self-acceptance and insight when we can gain a perspective on ourselves. It is not the universal tendency to under- or overestimate ourselves that is problematic; it is our need to defend that position. Stephen Mitchell (1986), in his early classic paper on narcissism, said, "Healthy narcissism reflects the same subtle dialectical balance between illusion and reality; illusions concerning oneself and others are generated, playfully enjoyed and relinquished in the face of disappointments. New illusions are continually created and dissolved" (p. 120).

Gender and narcissism in therapists

The few others writing on the subject of the therapist's needs and personality include Farber and Heifetz (1981) and Luchner et al. (2008). Luchner et al. say,

> [T]wo distinct forms of narcissism exist: a grandiose type that is exemplified by a heightened sense of self-worth and a covert type that is exemplified by a devalued sense of self-worth marked by timidity, inhibition and an overwhelming sense of failure rather than accomplishment. (p. 2)

On this point, I refer the reader to the previous chapter regarding our need to see the analyst as long-suffering. Luchner et al.'s definitions are more extreme, but one might argue that being infinitely patient and tolerant, with little room for anger or any strong negative feelings toward patients, represents a certain type of narcissistic ideal. In light of my previous comments on the changes occurring over time in the analytic persona due to culture and gender, I found these comments by Welt and Herron (1990) regarding gender differences to have been prescient. They say women are more concerned with relatedness than men, while men may feel compelled to protect their self-image by remaining cool and detached. They propose that women may be more sensitive to aggressive attacks and criticisms of their caretaking abilities.

These are 30-year-old generalizations, of course, and have to be considered as such. Were the aforementioned White, male, MD's more likely to fit this stereotype? I can easily think of many male analysts who do not resemble the "cool and detached" male therapists described by Welt and Herron, nor do they exemplify the grandiose type of narcissism described by Luchner et al.

As stated earlier in this volume, the emotional and cultural landscape of psychoanalysis is changing. Male psychoanalysts today are more likely to be psychologists or social workers—again attesting to the cultural and generational changes that have impacted analytic theory and practice. And they are as affected by the rise of attachment literature and the emphasis on the real relationship in treatment, as well as by their increasing numbers of female colleagues, teachers, and supervisors.

A thorny question is to what extent our rebellion against the arrogant, grandiose classical analyst stereotype has produced a new generation of those inclined toward *covert narcissism* as described by Luchner et al. Is the current debate over what is generous and kind, versus what is masochistic, a function of this newer analytic ideal? Has the new analytic persona become one of endless self-sacrifice and unpretentiousness? And to what extent does this ideal represent not a minimization of a narcissistic ideal, but rather a reaction formation to the old one? As Kravis (2013) points out,

> Analysts who rigidly eschew idealization are at risk for sinking into another kind of complacency. They might come to see themselves as highly evolved beings who have transcended the pedestrian gratifications of being admired for skill and expertise, and now live on a plane of great humility that has them floating above their narcissistically needy brethren. (p. 91)

As a woman, I am not anxious to ascribe some of the current weaknesses in theoretical and clinical preferences to the influence of female analysts. But if we recognize the significant positive impact of women on our ways of theorizing and practicing, we necessarily must also consider the weaknesses that may accompany that perspective. I think we cannot take credit for this humanizing of the analytic process without also considering some drawbacks to the emphasis, embraced now by both men and women, on mother–infant attachment styles and the need for unconditional acceptance.

Has the ascendance of self-psychology and relational psychoanalysis, along with the influence of women in psychoanalysis, created a greater sense of personal responsibility for treatment outcomes? Has our emphasis on attachment and affective attunement led us to this dual blind spot of feeling so responsible we feel compelled to defend against any internal or external charge of having erred? Is this part of why the whole subject of therapeutic error has virtually disappeared? In the case example below, I ponder one of my own errors.

The case of Jennifer

Jennifer, a 50ish business executive, had been in treatment with me for four years. In a testament to long-term treatment, she had made significant progress and our relationship was strong. She also faced and make or break situation in her life outside of treatment—the suicide attempt and psychiatric hospitalization of her teenage son.

For the first few years of treatment, she described herself as catering to the needs of her husband, a self-proclaimed entrepreneur who makes little money but spends a great deal. Obviously, part of the countertransference is that I have come to dislike the husband, who I have never met. It is not lost on me, however, that I dislike him *for Jennifer*, and that she has colluded with him over the years to create an unstable punitive environment where he critiques everyone constantly and flies into rages over the slightest disappointment (like one of the kids bringing home a B+ grade on a paper instead of an A).

Jennifer has always said she knows he is unreasonable and harsh. But she needed to believe his claim that he acted out of wanting only the best for his family and believing that high expectations were required for success. Jennifer began treatment, by the way, due to debilitating increases in her chronic anxiety and depression. She was not suicidal but found herself frequently wishing she was dead.

During the first few years of treatment, she was so anxious and depressed, in spite of her tremendous success in her chosen field, I knew not to even consider discussing the subject of verbal abuse by her husband. Whenever I asked her how she felt about his behavior, having clearly described it in a manner that could only be construed as verbal assault, she would beg off and say that he was doing his best and wanted the best for his family. Over time, I became frustrated with her position, because I was ready for her to make more progress and recognize what was really going on in her household. But whenever I broached this topic, I saw her brows furrow as she looked away from me. The breaking point for me came when her son's mental health deteriorated to the point of him starving himself and acting out at school.

As Jennifer described his behavior, which was becoming increasingly bizarre, I began to gently point out to her that she and her husband needed to get professional help for him. She discussed this with her husband and son, but they both concluded that it was not necessary. When she told me about the extremely harsh criticism her husband continued to level at him, I focused on him for a bit. But she was equally unprepared to acknowledge the damage her husband had done to her children and to her.

At the time, I was insufficiently aware of my own need to impose my view of reality on Jennifer. I feared the outcome if her son did not get help soon, and I took on too much responsibility for a possible horrific outcome. I was becoming very frustrated when she and her husband did nothing as he continued to deteriorate.

I do feel that my strong suggestions regarding getting treatment for him were appropriate to a point, but my repeatedly bringing it up was gratuitous. Jennifer's response to my frequent references to the troubling aspects of her son's behavior was to defensively brag about how brilliant he was (which was true) and what a prodigy he was on the piano (also true). I sat quietly judging her and her husband for their narcissism as they basked in their son's accomplishments while his mental health deteriorated. I know Jennifer saw the look on my face when she did this, and I began to realize that my attitude had turned negative, in spite of my affection and respect for Jennifer overall.

What I didn't fully appreciate at the time was how much of my own narcissism was at work in these repetitive failures to connect. In my mind, I knew what needed to happen and I felt frustrated and thwarted when I could not get Jennifer on board with my agenda.

It was only when Jennifer began to shut down, saying very little to me in most of her sessions (and missing more frequently than she needed to) that I realized I had driven her into retreat. As I observed her turning away from me, I became more motivated to examine my own behavior and motivations. In my mind, the simple fact that she had to flee the pressure I was putting on her says I was addressing my own needs rather than hers. I have said before that even if you are "right"—in this case, this boy didn't get treatment until he subsequently needed to be hospitalized—this should not be confused with doing what is therapeutic.

Luckily, I was able to change my attitude and work more closely with her, accepting that she was not ready to admit to the seriousness of her son's condition. I frankly told her that I realized I had been too critical and too impatient, which she acknowledged was true. I also began to be more accepting when she regaled me with her son's latest triumph. It was difficult for me to accept that I was helpless to change this scenario, but I was.

Eventually her son did attempt suicide and was admitted to the hospital for an extensive stay. I was relieved that his self-harm did not do any lasting damage, and Jennifer became more willing to discuss the reality of their family situation, including her role and her husband's. Her son's hospitalization broke through her defensive wish that he was just going through a rebellious stage and would be okay.

Following this extreme family crisis, Jennifer rose to the occasion, noting her own failures, especially her failure to protect her children from her husband's sadism. Equally as important, she reflected on her own motivations and needs to marry someone like him. She continued to build on this progress over time, and I was ultimately incredibly impressed with her insights and courage. When I reflect on my relationship with her, I remind myself that I easily could have ruined that treatment had I not come to my senses as she withdrew from me.

As I said, knowing that her son badly needed professional help, and also wanting her to stop taking abuse from her husband, initially motivated my interventions. But, over time, my interventions became more motivated by my frustrated needs to fix things and change Jennifer. Perhaps because of her many strengths, I thought she could handle the truth. But she was not ready. I was wrong in thinking she would never be if I didn't do more. And even now, I am surprised at how difficult it can be to identify overzealous interventions that are as much or more about me as they are about the patient. My lifelong identity as the family problem solver and "fixer" allows me to quickly and accurately assess situations and know what needs to happen. But it also sometimes results in me taking too much responsibility and attempting to control situations that I cannot. Accepting helplessness is not one of my strengths, but I noticeably feel better once I do.

As Jennifer approached termination and we revisited the trajectory of her treatment, I asked her this: "I am quite impressed not only with the level of insight you've acquired over the last year but also your ability to change your behavior. You don't seem to have any difficulty acknowledging the 'truths' both positive and negative, regarding yourself, your husband, and the family in general. What I want to know is, looking back to the time you began your therapy, do you feel that you always really knew the truth, but couldn't manage the feelings that accompanied it, or that you gradually came to see the truth over time?"

Jennifer looked me right in the eye and said, "The former. I knew the truth, but it terrified me. And I had no idea how I would ever make my way out of the mess I'd created. It was too overwhelming, so I always worked to counter it with the idea that I should think positive and everything would be okay. But, of course, it wasn't. My son's suicide attempt was the last straw." I think my greatest error with Jennifer is that I confused my accurate assessment that she knew the truth, with her being ready to bear it. And I am glad she was able to communicate her displeasure with me rather than simply leaving.

Langs (1973) says that every patient has a "tell," even when they are doing their best to protect the therapist by denying any anger or disapproval they may feel. I agree. Most patients have to look away when they are answering untruthfully, or answer in a weaker than normal voice, or defensively exaggerate the therapist's skill and devotion, or answer questions like "Are you angry with me?' with equivocal statements like "not really" or "I don't think so." Jennifer's way of dealing with me was to withdraw, which had been a long-time strategy for her.

It is not only conflict that we can ignore, of course. For myself, I have been equally oblivious at times to my patients' displaced expressions of love, admiration, or sexual attraction to me. In my attempts to eschew the narcissistic position of assuming one is the "love object," I have missed the opportunity to name their longings and desires related to me. Did I really not want to be the love object or did I want it so much I had to deny it?

Again, this speaks to the tension, as named by many of the authors cited in this chapter, that exists between accepting and defending an idealized view versus a denigrated one, a need to rescue versus a need to distance, and a need to be needed versus a need to be free and autonomous. As Mitchell (1986) said, the answer is not to transcend these feelings. We cannot. The answer lies in our self-awareness and our capacity to see ourselves for who we really are without undue guilt and shame.

Conclusion

A largely unexplored area of inquiry in psychoanalysis revolves around the analyst's ongoing, and essential, narcissistic vulnerability. If we cannot be wounded by our patients, how involved are we? If they do not have the power to hurt us, how important can they be? It seems that our "work ego" or analytic persona has left little room for the natural vulnerability that results from emotional engagement. We endorse the former, but not the latter.

One of the legacies of classical analysis remains "the perfectly analyzed analyst." I have proposed that we tend to err in the direction of either blaming ourselves excessively when the treatment process is stalled or unsuccessful, or defending against this superego assault by convincing ourselves that everything we do is "grist for the mill" and therefore acceptable or even desirable.

Understanding how these unrealistic expectations evolved from being the family caregiver can help analysts accept both their own human flaws and limitations, as well as their patients'. It can also help them to more deeply appreciate their natural empathic abilities, curiosity, commitment, and other character traits that serve them and their patients. In the next chapter, I will discuss how our reluctance to acknowledge the ways in which we wish to influence our patients and our discomfort with conflict work in tandem to effect the treatment.

References

Coen, S. (2007). Narcissistic temptations to cross boundaries and how to manage them. *Journal of the American Psychoanalytic Association, 55,* 1169–1190.

Chused, J. (2012). The analyst's narcissism. *Journal of the American Psychoanalytic Association, 60,* 899–915.

Eagle, M. (2007). Psychoanalysis and its critics. *Psychoanalytic Psychology, 24,* 10–24.

Farber, B. A., & Heifetz, L. J. (1981). The satisfactions and stresses of psychotherapeutic work: A factor analytic study. *Professional Psychology, 12,* 621–630.

Finell, J. (1985). Narcissistic problems in analysts. *International Journal of Psychoanalysis, 66,* 433–445.

Frommer, M. S. (2013). When the analyst's protected space is breached: Commentary on Paper by Stephanie R. Brody. *Psychoanalytic Dialogues, 23,* 59–71.

Gill, M. M. (1984). Transference: A change in conception or only in emphasis? *Psychoanalytic Inquiry, 4,* 489–523.

Greenberg, J. (2001). The analyst's participation: A new look. *Journal of the American Psychoanalytic Association, 49,* 358–381.

Hirsch, I. (2008). *Coasting in the countertransference: Conflicts of self-interest between analyst and patient.* New York: The Analytic Press.

Hirsch, I. (2011). Narcissism, envy and the analyst's envy. *American Journal of Psychoanalysis, 71,* 363–369.

Hirsch, I. (2014). Narcissism, mania and analysts' envy of patients. *Psychoanalytic Inquiry, 34,* 408–420.

Kilborne, B. (2007). Shame, empathy and analytic training. *The Candidate, 2,* 1–4

Kohut, H. (1971). *The analysis of the self.* Madison, CT: International Universities Press, Inc.

Kravis, N. (2013). The analyst's hatred of analysis. *Psychoanalytic Quarterly, 82,* 89–114.

Kuchuck, S. (2009). Do ask, do tell? Narcissistic need as a determinant of analyst self-disclosure. *Psychoanalytic Review, 96,* 1007–1024.

Langs, R. (1973). *The technique of psychoanalytic psychotherapy* (Vol. 2). New York: Aronson.

Little, M. (1951). Countertransference and the patient's response to it. *International Journal of Psychoanalysis, 32,* 240–254.

Livingston, M. (2003). Vulnerability, affect and depth in group psychotherapy. *Psychoanalytic Inquiry, 23,* 646–677.

Luchner, A. F., Mose, C. J., Mirsalimi, H., & Jones, R. A. (2008). Maintaining boundaries in psychotherapy: Covert narcissistic personality characteristics and psychotherapists. *Psychotherapy: Theory, Research, Practice, Training, 45*, 1–14.

Mitchell, S. (1986). The wings of Icarus: Illusion and the problem of narcissism. *Contemporary Psychoanalysis, 22*, 107–132.

Pinsky, E. (2011). The Olympian delusion. *Journal of the American Psychoanalytic Association, 59*, 351–375.

Pulver, S. (1970). Narcissism: The term and the concept. *Journal of the American Psychoanalytic Association, 18*, 319–341.

Seligson. A. G. (1992). The narcissistic therapist meets a narcissistic patient. *Journal of Contemporary Psychotherapy, 22*, 221–225.

Sussman, M. (1992). *A curious calling.* New York: Aronson.

Welt, S. R., & Herron, W. G. (1990). *Narcissism and the psychotherapist.* New York: Guilford.

Wilson, M. (2003). The analyst's desire and the problem of narcissistic resistances. *Journal of the American Psychoanalytic Association, 51*, 71–99.

Wilson, M. (2013). Desire and responsibility: The ethics of countertransference experience. *The Psychoanalytic Quarterly, 82*, 435–476.

Wink, P. (1996). Two faces of narcissism. *Journal of Personality and Social Psychology, 61*, 590–597.

Wolf, E. S. (1988). *Treating the self: Elements of clinical self psychology.* New York: Guilford.

Part II

The analyst as clinician

Chapter 4

Conflict and negative countertransference

Psychoanalysts today still look for unconsciously determined events and still place great emphasis on self-awareness. However, the twin notions of conflict and the analyst's role as knowledgeable facilitator of that conflict have faded into the background. Dent and Christian (2019) reported that within the pages of the *Journal of the American Psychoanalytic Association*, the word *conflict* appeared with the greatest frequency in 1987 and has suffered a steady decline since. Do psychoanalysts no longer believe in conflict as an essential aspect of human experience? Is it truly no longer the centerpiece of analytic treatment? I think the answer to these questions is complicated.

While references to conflict have undeniably decreased, I think it likely that similar research on the word "enactment" would reveal a corresponding increase in usage over the same period of time. Enactment is conflict personified, but it is heavily weighted toward the interpersonal rather than the intrapsychic. And, perhaps more importantly, co-experiencing it with the patient is increasingly seen as the "accidental encounter"—unplanned and nondeliberate. It is not part of any formal theory of conflict resolution nor therapeutic action.

In line with the overall thesis of this book, to what extent has conflict also been de-emphasized in favor of the concept of becoming the "good enough" object? And to what extent have we, once again, taken slices of different theoretical approaches and combined them, not just to integrate the best of what each has to offer but also to conform to our preferred personal style and overall psychological make-up? What both classical and two-person theories have in common is the analyst's reluctance to admit to mutual influence and the inevitable conflicts that ensue.

Let us begin with a brief overview of the uses of conflict in hopes of gaining some insight into how it has fallen into disfavor and also how it continues as a basic tenet of analytic work.

A brief history of conflict

Freudian analysis revolved around the assumption of internal conflict as *the* problem to be addressed. Innate drives potentially at odds with the environment, as well as internal values (e.g., sex and aggression), generated these conflicts. It was the analyst's job to interpret conflicts and identify how they were expressed in the patient's life. The patient's tendency to "forget" the basis for his or her conflict even after it had been identified in the treatment setting inspired Freud to coin the term "resistance." He said that resistance was not the act of an uncooperative patient, but rather a natural tendency to re-forget that which we were pushing out of awareness to begin with. Resistance was commonly due to unbearable guilt and shame over ambivalent ties to loved ones, as well as sexual desires. The analyst understood that repetition was inevitable and that interpretations must be made again and again.

Conflict with the analyst was secondary, occurring not because the analyst had contributed to it, but rather because the patient's transference created it. The analyst's task was to remain above the fray and interpret that the patient was projecting his own issues, and the characteristics of his parents, onto the analyst.

Engaging actively in the present with the patient as he or she played out their early-established conflicts was not seriously considered. Neither, of course, was the analyst's contributions to the relationship as a real person with flaws and blind spots of his own. Thus, the classical analyst, while making the patient's internal conflicts front and center, did not pursue any substantial discussion of what was going on interpersonally between them. Ego psychology and modern conflict theory, likewise, did not acknowledge the impact of the treatment as a subjective relationship with its own unique potential for conflict.

Christian (2015) says,

> *Modern conflict theory*, a term that Abend (1994; in Brenner, 2008) coined to denote Brenner's important modifications of classical ego psychology, emphasizes the ubiquity of conflict, of unconscious fantasy, and compromise formations as the essence of mental functioning, including that of the analyst. Yet in his writings, Brenner gave little importance to the role of countertransference or subjectivity in the therapeutic process. (p. 610)

Therefore, even as Freudian theory was morphing into ego psychology and modern conflict theory, the analyst as a person, deeply involved in the patient's conflicts, was not a focus of clinical analysis. Psychoanalysis has come a long way since then. Although a history of the two-person approach goes beyond the scope of this chapter (see Aron, 1996), suffice it to say that a huge paradigm shift occurred with the rise of interpersonal, object relations, self-psychology, intersubjective, and relational theories.

Relational theory

People frequently ask, "What happened to the concept of conflict in psychoanalysis?" Relational theory, in particular, has been criticized for lacking a theoretical framework for conflict. Relational analyst Adrienne Harris (2005), in her attempt to address this issue, notes, "the exercise involved in writing this article—to think about conflict from a relational perspective—has been challenging and demanding because relational theorists have not made conflict a central, explicit focus of interest" (p. 267).

In place of the Freudian focus on intrapsychic conflict, Relational theory, in particular, all but discarded traditional drive theory in favor of a theory of the "drive to connect"—the innate need to create and maintain relationships. Rather than seeing the patient as tortured by his sexual and aggressive impulses, Relational founders Jay Greenberg and Stephen Mitchell (1988) made relationships the primary focus of life and of treatment. They saw our conflicts as existing in proportion to the thwarting of our striving to be healthily related to others. We are in conflict, not essentially with ourselves, but rather with others in our environment. As Aron (1996) noted,

> Relational theorists have in common an interest in the intrapsychic as well as the interpersonal, but *the intrapsychic is seen as constituted largely by the internalization of interpersonal experience* mediated by the *constraints* imposed by biologically organized templated and delimiters. (p. 16, emphasis added)

The overarching theme states that all manner of symptoms and problems can arise due to a lack of affirmation and constructive emotional engagement. These are the primary concerns of the Relational analyst, not sex and aggression.

The focus on patterns established in early childhood remains intact, but Gabbard (1997) notes that the two-person approach dramatically altered how we conceive of these patterns. He says that with the increasing interest in affect and attachment the analysand's recurring patterns were defined more as the result of early mother-infant interactions: "*The notion of intrapsychic conflicts faded into the background as the emphasis was placed on interpersonal conflicts as primary*" (p. 21, emphasis added).

Going even further, Busch (2005) criticizes the approach taken by those treating trauma patients, saying that the interpsychic aspect of repression is consistently overlooked. He says, "The role of ongoing intrapsychic conflicts in keeping feelings hidden tends to be ignored" (p. 28). However, it was never Mitchell's intention to weaken the position of conflict in relational theory. Rather, his goal was to reframe it.

Interestingly, Mitchell's (1988) own declarations regarding the place of conflict in Relational theory are infrequently discussed. Contrary to popular opinion, he saw conflict as central to his theory. He felt that assigning conflict to drive theory alone was an error and did not represent his relational theory and its clinical applications. He wanted analysts to understand that even though his theoretical take on conflict differed from classical theory, he remained committed to a model that included it. Rather than sexual and aggressive drives as the basis for conflict, he saw the fear of losing important relationships as primary.

In what I see as a relational take on what Freud labeled the Oedipal conflict, Mitchell (1988) says our conflicts emanate from familial relationships and the fear of losing them: "[T]he universality of conflicts between and among different relationships and identifications; ties and loyalties to one parent are, to some extent, inevitably experienced as (and in reality, may very well be) a threat to ties and loyalties to the other" (p. 160). He also made it clear that he saw conflict as universal and ubiquitous, stating that "... *conflict is inherent in relatedness*" (p. 160).

Thus Mitchell establishes that relationships, from the very beginning, are a source of both needed emotional supplies and of conflict. He specifically references the developing child's awareness that what might please one parent may not please another. So who is the patient to be when in their joint presence? And is he or she being disloyal when feeling more aligned with one parent over the other? I would add to this early constellation the much-neglected early conflicts imbedded in sibling rivalry. Wanting to defeat one's siblings, but not harm them, provides fertile ground for years of both internal and external conflict. Mitchell was well aware of these universal conflicts and wanted relational theory and practice to incorporate them.

So why has Mitchell's important contributions on conflict been so overlooked? Perhaps, in part, because of the popularity of Winnicott's work, which is at odds with Mitchell's stance. Winnicott has been lionized over the last 25 years to the point that the accuracy of his views is rarely challenged. If Winnicott said it, it must be true. But to what extent is the idealization of Winnicott based on the shared early experience of analysts?

Affirming a major tenet of this book, Winnicott openly admitted to the burden he felt from having felt compelled to heal his depressed mother. But neither he nor those who are devoted to his work have given consideration to how this background served to both inform and limit his theory and clinical interventions. Did his openly declared misery in response to his mother's demands not create conflict for him? Was he not ambivalent toward her? Was his desire to be the caretaker of his patients a result of his longing to be taken care of himself? Did he not avoid conflict with his patients as a repetition of his perceived need to protect his mother from his anger and unhappiness?

Although he did not concern himself with Winnicott's motivations, Mitchell was not reluctant to challenge the ideas of Winnicott and other object relations theorists in his early writing. He attributed the neglect of conflict to their influence on how relational concepts were implemented. Mitchell (1984) referred to the unwelcome comparison of the mother–infant dyad to the analytic dyad as "the developmental tilt." He very plainly stated that the neglect of conflict is not inherent in the relational approach, but rather something that gradually occurred as a result of the implementation of developmental theories within relational psychoanalysis. He felt strongly that the neglect of conflict significantly limited the contributions of relational theory.

It had been so long since I first read *Relational Concepts in Psychoanalysis* (1988) that I was quite surprised by Mitchell's criticisms of Winnicott and others who anchored their clinical and theoretical approach to developmental deficits. In fact, I had forgotten that Mitchell had ever taken this stand. If I am not alone, there is a good reason for this. In ensuing years, the attachment literature and affect literature became both prominent and compelling. Mitchell gradually changed his views, agreeing that the impact of mother-infant attachment was a core concept that impacted the analyst–patient relationship. His later writing basically dropped any reference to the "developmental tilt" in favor of incorporating important attachment and affect research. The following quote from him demonstrates how strong his one-time objections to seeing the patient as an infant were:

> Some analytic work done under the aegis of object relations theory via the developmental tilt is thus marred by a collusion between the patient's fantasy and the analyst's theory; the patient is jointly viewed as an exquisitely delicate and brittle infant to be handled in just the right fashion by a uniquely sensitive caretaker, leading to a splitting of the transference and a removal of the analysis from the world of real people, from which it never returns. (p. 497)

His incisive commentary explicitly acknowledges that the patient may well have fantasies about being held, re-parented, or rescued in some fashion by the idealized analyst-parent. Yet it is this siren call that he specifically warns against, just as Searles had more than 20 years earlier. Mitchell worried precisely about the tendency for therapists to get caught up in being the *uniquely sensitive caregiver*, fearing that the patient's negative feelings would ultimately be forced underground, never to resurface.

Mitchell's final psychoanalytic book, *Relationality: From Attachment to Intersubjectivity* (2000), contains no mention of his former objections to the influence of object relations theory on relational theory and technique. His references to Winnicott are purely as literature review, absent any comment about his clinical choices and his impact on the field. Wachtel (2017) discussed the controversy over whether or not Michell truly abandoned his early views on the developmental tilt. Wachtel's opinion is that he did not, simply because it wasn't inherently demanded. He could integrate attachment research without doing so.

Although I understand Wachtel's point regarding Mitchell's characteristic willingness to embrace and integrate new ideas and research, which he clearly did, I'm not sure this really addresses the issue. There is no dispute that Mitchell was impacted by the research on attachment and affective development in early childhood and ceased to express his negative critique of the emphasis on the adult patient's experience in infancy. But, as previously stated, and illustrated in quotes from Mitchell's work, I believe his issue with Winnicott and other object relations thinkers had more to do with what Mitchell perceived as their influence on the *implementation* of relational theory, rather than his opinion of the importance of early attachments.

Mitchell did not object to placing importance on the idea that many patients had suffered early in their lives from a lack of adequate parenting—rather, he objected to a *clinical stance* that de-emphasized conflict in favor of a narrow focus on the analyst as reparative parent. It seems to me that this stands alone, regardless of his greater appreciation for early attachment issues. I make this point, in part, because my own current views are very similar to Mitchell's early views regarding the emphasis on early deficits.

My own theoretical trajectory

Ironically, my own views have been shaped inversely to Mitchell's. I began my career steeped in the work of Bowlby (1969, 1973),

Mahler et al. (1975), Fairbairn (1954), Guntrip (1969), and Winnicott (1960), having written my doctoral dissertation on separation anxiety. I also learned about affect theory in a graduate class where Silvan Tomkins was a guest lecturer. Thus, I was influenced by these writings very early in my career development, and I struggled to incorporate them with the ego psychology and self-psychology that dominated the analytic terrain during those years. Later, I went on to research affect theory and neuroscience, excited by the work of people like Schore (1994, 2001a, 2001b), Stern (1985), LeDoux (1994), and others. In 1998, I presented a paper on the importance of affective communication in treatment at the annual Division 39 meetings.

Just as I was beginning my clinical career, Winnicott's work was gaining in popularity. This was soon to be followed by what might be called the "trauma movement." Soon, many analytic conferences were peppered with case reports by relational analysts treating trauma survivors who had outsized needs and desperate desires to be reparented by their analysts. The emphasis in analytic work soon shifted to ways of responding to these difficult patients with what is often called "extreme empathy," characterized by the willingness to provide a heretofore unacceptable standard of availability at every level.

Calls in the middle of the night, sessions added on demand, the acceptance of graphic sexual talk, and a high tolerance for verbal abuse became more frequently reported. Interventions that would have previously be considered as boundary crossings, or even violations, have become more acceptable, often viewed as self-sacrificing instances of taking radical responsibility (as stated in Chapter 2). For myself, these lapses in the treatment frame have always seemed counterintuitive. Trauma generated by emotional and physical abuse is inherently a violation of boundaries.

Although trauma patients may well seek the fluid boundaries they have always known, is this not part of what needs to change? The traditional thought on keeping good boundaries is that it provides needed structure and safety, allowing the patient to surrender more easily during the prescribed limits of the relationship. Do traumatized patients need this less than other patients? This concept does not really make sense to me.

I have not heard any convincing argument for this lack of boundaries, other than that trauma patients need "special" attention due to the damage they suffered. This begs the question: What is the basis for developmental tilt theories and/or interventions? Are they truly responsive to the patient's needs, or do developmental deficit theories allow the analyst to identify with the patient who lacked early nurturing, thereby bypassing the threat of seeing him as a voracious adult?

In previous chapters, I have stated that we naturally avoid conflict because we were not allowed to be in conflict with our own parents. Our job was to soothe and comfort, not object and confront. Winnicott sadly noted that as a child he made his "living" by trying to keep his depressed mother alive. This is not a situation that promotes an interpersonal challenge. Again, do his ideas about the "good enough mother" and the need for "holding" find a home with so many analysts because they speak to the reparative and nurturing function that we all learned to perform at a young age? And do we overidentify with our suffering patients, wanting more to soothe and comfort them rather than confront them?

Hirsch (1987) said this about Winnicott's approach:

> Winnicott views the analyst as a totally loving figure. Even when the analyst hates, he is hating objectively and doing it for carefully planned therapeutic reasons. Winnicott believes that his good mother can resist being a bad mother. He maintains a good parent position and doesn't become enmeshed as a bad parent. (p. 214)

Over time, I became increasingly uncomfortable with this scenario. Not long ago, I listened to a panel at a Division 39 meeting where a 55-year-old patient, seen five times per week, was described as decompensating into an infantile state, curled up in the fetal position on the analyst's floor. She also contacted the analyst frequently outside of sessions with phone calls and emails. As I listened to this presentation of what was considered a successful ongoing treatment, my stomach started to churn.

The supervisors on this case—both well-known senior analysts—praised the presenting therapist for her "heroic" efforts with this very disturbed woman and applauded the sacrifices she made in the interest of helping her to work through her childhood trauma. Since the case was an ongoing one, there was no reported outcome. But I couldn't, quite frankly, imagine a good one. To my mind, the patient was being encouraged to regress to the extent that she could barely function. (She didn't work.) Her extreme dependence on her analyst rendered her life outside of treatment irrelevant. Even worse, the more concessions she received from her analyst, the more she requested. It is hard for me to conceive of this situation as therapeutic.

My current re-reading of Mitchell's views on the "developmental tilt" proved to be an affirming experience. I was pleasantly surprised to see how similar his 1988 views on the subject are to mine now. No doubt I integrated his views into mine decades ago when I first read his book. I wonder what he might say now, 20 years after his untimely death, about the clinical course the relational model has taken. The more I talk with analysts and therapists, the more concerned I am about the pursuit of harmony within the analytic dyad, as well as the excuses made for patient's unacceptable behavior. What follows is an example.

The case of Robert

I recently supervised an analyst who was seeing a patient I will call Robert. Robert had a history of losing jobs and alienating everyone around him because of his outlandish, abusive rages. He formed an intense, adoring transference to his analyst, telling her repeatedly how much he loved her and was in love with her. He was fiercely intelligent and read the analytic literature, even though he was a software engineer in Silicon Valley. He did so in the interests of entering and navigating her world, but also to acquire the ability to critique and intimidate her. He routinely pled for her to acknowledge that she, too, loved him. When she did not, he would send her expletive-ridden, misogynistic, verbal assaults.

To her mind, he was getting better because he now reserved his rages primarily for her and functioned much better in the world. I might have agreed, had he not become so obsessive about her and increased his demands for a proclamation of love from her. She had indulged him with numerous extra sessions, phone calls and emails, all of which fueled his desires and fantasy that one day they would be lovers.

The analyst in question knew things had gotten out of control, yet had great difficulty setting appropriate limits with this patient. When he sobbed and told her she was the only one who understood and accepted him, she melted. She viewed his rages as offensive, even frightening at times, but needed to see him as a frustrated, raging infant who could not always control himself. Her attempts to set better limits with him, as she worked to defuse this escalating tension, resulted in abusive rants and accusations of abandonment and betrayal. They were either basking in the glow of their intense feelings for each other or attempting to recover from equally intense ruptures. The focus of the treatment was almost exclusively "the relationship."

What became clear to me in working with this therapist was, first, that she loved "being loved" by this extremely bright patient who was laser-focused on knowing and possessing her, and second, that she felt guilt and shame when her own anger flared up. Defending against her unacceptable negative feelings towards this patient, she excused his inexcusable behavior, ascribing it to his own traumatic history. To my mind, she had slowly become immersed in a mutual "love cure" fantasy with him, as well as losing sight of the fact that in treatment, as in life, "what you permit, you promote."

Certainly, there was plenty of conflict in this relationship. Robert's perpetual rages about the asymmetry and his need to be openly loved by his analyst follow a common clinical trajectory. Yet, clinical vignettes rarely focus on the analyst's contributions to this scenario and equally rarely entail any expression of frustration or anger. The conflict between analyst and patient under these circumstances is both intrapsychic and interpersonal—fraught with longing, pathos, fear, and guilt. Mitchell (1997) cites Racker's classic work on how patient and analyst stimulate each other's primitive impulses and that our early longings and anxieties cannot be analyzed away. It's more a matter of when, rather than if, the patient stimulates us in this way. Mitchell says, "Thus, for Racker, the patient's projections are not received by the analyst's suspending his own memories and desires; the patient's projections are received by discovering which of one's own memories and desires have been stirred up" (pp. 115–116). I wish Mitchell could have elaborated more on this important point regarding the analyst's own inevitable primitive countertransference. He and Racker effectively point to the existence of these feelings not as an anomaly, but rather as part of the human condition. The analyst's overdeveloped superego and need to be seen as good often interferes with our ability to recognize the triggering of our own memories and desires, let alone judge how they are impacting the treatment. To the extent that we are aware of these feelings, they too often are rapidly replaced with guilt and shame. Celenza (2010) comments on how the analyst's excessive guilt and sense of responsibility influence the treatment.

> If the analytic superego is too strong, the analyst may respond to this pressure in a variety of undesirable ways … One of the most common is the attitude of reparation and atonement: What can I do to compensate the poor patient for the terrible suffering that he is going through, since some of it is really my fault. (p. 8)

Learning to recognize how our own fears and desires lay in wait, ready to be stimulated in a heartbeat by our patients, is critical to the analytic endeavor. Again, this is not possible without greater self-acceptance and minimizing of guilt and shame. Though it may be tempting to believe that most of us do find a way to deal with our negative responses to patients, the research begs to differ. Wolf et al. (2017) report

> In our study, we failed to encounter a single instance in which a difficult client's hostility and negativism were successfully confronted or resolved … therapists' negative responses to difficult clients are far more common and for more intractable than has been generally recognized. (p. 954)

I think this points to both our fears, our guilt, and also to the simple fact that high-level management of analyst conflicts with patients is not taught. As with many other aspects of technique, our preferred stance is relying on intuition and spontaneity. But I strongly disagree, in that conflict resolution in any type of relationship requires a certain skill set that needs to be learned and practiced.

And if I am correct regarding therapists' formative years spent *avoiding conflict* in our families of origin, therapist training necessarily needs to address this perspective as something to be factored in and even overcome. The unique empathic abilities and sensitivities that created our special role in our families and, ultimately, our vocational choice are a strength; our need to soothe and comfort others while avoiding conflict is not. Difficult patients are "difficult," in large part, because they frustrate us, thwart us, and most importantly, stimulate our primitive rage. The only solution to this clinical conundrum is for therapists to actually embrace their rage and desire to retaliate against the patient, rather than withdraw or embrace extreme empathy as a reaction formation. Welt and Herron (1990) note our tendency to defend against our anger, asserting that we are often afraid to experience it and rationalize this by saying it would not be useful for the patient: "The merits or demerits of such revelations aside, it would seem that the main issue is that the therapist is afraid of losing control because the patients may return the anger, thus stirring up the therapist's residual rage" (p. 9).

Failure to address conflict

Earlier in this volume, I laid out the case for not only our conflict avoidance, but for our need to see ourselves as transcending human nature. We have expectations for perfection that deny reality. Once we centered our theory and practice on therapy as a relationship, we had the perfect opportunity to explore the inevitable conflicts inherent in any relationship, as Mitchell noted. Why hasn't this new perspective on conflict, placing the interpersonal as the jumping off point for all conflict, produced a wealth of literature in its own right? As more and more of the interactions between analyst and patient came to be defined as "mutual," somehow the mutual desires to both connect and maintain autonomy, as well as maintain homeostasis (Aron, 1991), failed to produce the expected conversations and innovations.

What gets lost in our conversations about mutuality is the reality of mutual *influence*—not in the sense that we all ultimately effect each other (which, of course we do), but in the sense that from day one we are concerned with our own self-interest and are motivated to maintain our own psychic well-being, even if it brings us into conflict with others. This is true of our patients and ourselves. Slavin and Kriegman (1998) point out our reluctance in attributing conflict to this natural state of competing needs. They say we prefer other explanations:

> We believe that all analytic traditions overemphasize the extent to which differences in the subjectivities of patient and analyst result from either instinctual clashes, relational failures, or the accidents of an imperfect world. Rather, intersubjective disjunctions are often ultimately rooted in genuine conflicts of interest. In a variety of ways, it is conflicting interests that generate the continuing (self-interested) efforts at *mutual* influence that can be found within most therapeutic communications, and these conflicting interests are, inevitably, deceptively hidden within all versions of analytic technique. (p. 253)

I think Slavin and Kriegman make an excellent point: We have never focused on the natural conflicts that arise in any relationship, including the analytic one, in part because it would necessitate the examination of our own needs, desires, and shortcomings. Rather than increasing our self-awareness on these issues, it appears that we have preferred to go in the opposite direction. We not only avoid discussions of both our natural human tendencies and our personal flaws but we also have done the same in relation to our patients. They are increasingly seen as innocent victims in an interpersonal world that has let them down, and we are increasingly seen as the paradigms of virtue who can provide our patients with a better experience that will restore them. This "parentified" role for the analyst risks creating an expectation that neither analyst nor patient can meet. I think we need to find a way to retain the valuable insights and perspectives we have gleaned from the attachment literature, while integrating it with the reality of innate self-interest and the knowledge that even the best of us are flawed.

The intense emphasis on the mother–child relationship as one to be relived in treatment has resulted in interventions aimed at reducing conflict in favor of empathic attunement. However, the need for the mother and child to be as in sync as often as possible to facilitate the infant's early development is not a perfect model for analytic treatment. It is our dark sides, regardless of the source, that we struggle to accept and need to make peace with in treatment.

Thus, my argument is not with integrating the attachment literature into analytic theory and practice. Rather, it is what I see as an overemphasis on early attachments. As others have pointed out (e.g., Sperry, 2011), our development is not cast in stone at the end of the early attachment period, in spite of the establishment of attachment styles. And our needs and desires are certainly not the same. I think part of the attraction of the mother-infant model is that, ironically, it provides some of the same protective emotional distance formerly provided by the "transference" model. Neither of these conceptualizations provides a context for two mature individuals encountering each other with all their varied strengths as well as vulnerabilities.

As stated previously, the relational school is attempting to address some of these excesses and overemphasis on the mother–infant mode and to address Mitchell's point about development throughout the life cycle. Slochower (2018) says, "We've largely ignored models (e.g., Erickson, 1950; Kohut, 1971) that extend the developmental arc or developmental needs for attunement and repair beyond childhood" (p. 18).

I agree. Yet while acknowledging the limitations of a narrow focus on very early childhood when treating adult patients, the above quote reveals an ongoing concern with needs for "attunement and repair"—with no attention paid to the need to work through conflicts, either intrapsychic or interpersonal. There is little discussion of the increasing capacity for self-observation and an accompanying new perspective on others that is typically associated with adolescence. Parents are quick to note the frequency with which formerly adoring children turn into disappointed and critical teenagers, endlessly finding fault with them. Yet somehow this common wisdom has not made its way into relational theory, in spite of it being a natural segue from early childhood issues.

A burgeoning sense of autonomy lays the groundwork for deidealization and conflict with the analyst. I am not denying the continuing need for affirmation and empathy throughout the life span, as noted by Kohut (1971). But to emphasize this over the growing need for autonomy, and the conflict likely to arise from that need, does not do much to forward a developmental model for treatment. I doubt that seeing the patient as a damaged adult is going to provide a major corrective to seeing him as a damaged child.

The analyst's false self

Wilson (2013) speaks frankly about our denial of having our own agenda as treatment begins. He talks about our *analytic desires*, noting that such awareness is crucial to a successful treatment. My casual conversation with clinicians has readily revealed their awareness of wanting to influence patients from the very beginning, and also feeling some anxiety regarding how the patient might influence them. These ideas are often nascent and unformulated early on, but the gnawing feeling in the gut is there. Over time, the inherent struggle to influence each other becomes more recognizable.

I recall treating a very aggressive patient very early in my career who I was determined to understand and soothe. I believed if I was good enough and empathic enough, she would relax and begin to engage in a more productive and calm manner. My implicit goal was to transform her into a saner, more relaxed person.

What I soon realized was that the more attached she was to me and the safer she felt with me, the more demanding and aggressive she became. The reader may say, "Well, of course, that was the transference.". But knowing these things intellectually and navigating them personally are very different propositions—especially as a neophyte therapist. What goes unacknowledged, or is acknowledged only with shame, is how much we desire, in Wilson's terms, to change the people who come to us for treatment. Certainly, the more the patient is seeking these changes, the better the outcome.

But often we have an agenda that the patient does not. Sometimes this is related to timing, other times to the issue itself. And, because we are only human, we feel thwarted, frustrated, and eventually, angry when we are denied this influence by our patients. Likewise, they enter the treatment situation with a need to preserve themselves with a corresponding need to influence us. As much as my aggressive patient pleaded for my help, she continued to demand an impossible degree of reciprocity. When this was not forthcoming, nothing less would do other than for me to equally suffer her hopelessness and despair.

One day, in a rather startling moment, I was struck by the reality that she and I were endlessly working to defend our own realities and change each other. This insight was quickly followed by the realization that she was winning. Rather than the sessions ending with her being more self-aware and calmer, they were ending with me feeling frustrated, powerless, and angry. I discussed this case in *The Power of Countertransference* (Maroda, 1991), noting that I could only break free from this impasse when I admitted these feelings to myself and found a constructive way to express them to my patient.

Because of our need to deny self-interest, which flies in the face of our preferred self-sacrificing persona, we tend to create a therapeutic relationship that inevitably becomes false in its very essence. I say "false" because at those moments when the analyst is denying his attempts to influence the patient, he is generating a false narrative. As this denial of power-seeking and wishing to influence takes hold in the treatment, both sides can devolve into deception and a well-intentioned but doomed attempt to keep the relationship moving along.

The analyst or therapist can recognize this state, in part, because it usually produces a sense of uneasiness inside the therapist, with feelings of inadequacy creeping up as time goes on. The therapist feels like a failure, in part, because at some level of consciousness, she knows that she is not addressing the patient's needs, or her own, in a direct and honest manner. Rather, she is increasingly aware of cloud of uncertainty and confusion enveloping the relationship for as long as the conflict avoidance continues.

I believe that new therapists are particularly prone to feeling like imposters because they have little to no instruction in how to recognize, accept, and facilitate the normal conflicts inherent in the therapeutic relationship. And they tend to feel terribly guilty about their negative feelings toward their patients, particularly if the patient has suffered much in life. When the patient is also "suing for love" (Nunberg, 1934), anguishing over not being as important to the analyst as the analyst is to her, the analyst predictably feels sad and often guilty.

Celenza (2007) reminds us that the asymmetry of the relationship also creates its own unique brand of conflict and power struggles.

> From the outset, the analyst must withstand (by holding the tension) the analysand's pressure to disempower him or her. This is the pressure derived from the asymmetric distribution of attention and the analysand's attempts to ameliorate the humiliating consequences of it. In this regard, it is important that the analyst not feel undue guilt about the power inherent in the structured asymmetry of the analytic relationship. (p. 292)

I think she makes a good point in that facilitating conflict is not always active or overt. It can consist of simple quiet understanding of the patient's need to resist the analyst's influence. Negotiating the inherent mutual desires for power and influence does not necessarily suggest confrontation, although at times that will be necessary. Rather, the acceptance of separate realities and needs creates a space for creative recognition, even if that is nothing more than guilt-free silence. Again, Celenza (2010) provides some incisive comments regarding the analyst's guilt and resulting defensive maneuvers: "One of the most common is the attitude of reparation and atonement: What can I do to compensate the poor patient for the terrible suffering that he is going through, since some of it is really my fault" (p. 8).

When the analyst does not accept his or her own natural desires for power, influence, and even the need to keep the patient at bay sometimes, the result can be stultifying. When each side joins in this *mutual denial*, pacifying each other but not getting to the heart of what is really going on, mutual boredom, a sense of helplessness, and finally, frustration and anger emerge. When this continues over time, what inevitably follows is enactment (a topic I take up in depth in Chapter 5). Given the building up of tension between analyst and patient that I have described, it is not surprising that enactment comes as a relief, no matter how difficult or painful. The problem is whether or not waiting for enactment is the optimal clinical stance or an abdication of responsibility for facilitating constructive conflict. But in order to do this, I believe we need to first recognize and accept that we are, in fact, seeking to influence the patient, and that this represents a prosocial and desirable stance. I have long maintained that prosocial power seeking is an integral part of what we do and that out of fear of unseemly manipulation of the patient, we remain in denial of that pursuit.

Again, it seems evident that women are uniquely averse to seeing themselves as power seeking (Maroda, 2004), and thus the increased aversion to authority and influence in psychoanalysis may be related to the increasing influence of women in the profession. (As I pointed out earlier in this volume, I believe women are also responsible for the humanizing of psychoanalysis and the recognition of the importance of affect.)

Accepting that the very nature of our work involves power, and that this is not at odds with our commitment to acting in the patient's interest, could go a long way in exploring this issue productively. Power does not have to be a dirty word. The very definition of power describes the impact we wish to have on our patients. In her synthesis of the literature, Dunbar (2015) concludes,

> Despite the many definitions of power that exist in the interpersonal literature, scholars from diverse fields are converging on the definition of power generally as the capacity to produce intended effects, and in particular, the ability to influence the behavior of another person. (p. 2)

Perhaps we are so averse to the concept of influence because we know that our self-interest must play some part in this. Slavin and Kriegman (1998) additionally examine our excessive preoccupation with being empathic as a defense against the analyst's self-interest, which can generate pseudo-empathy and deception. They describe consistent empathy as "unnatural," noting that therapists may "use the empathic stance to remain defensively hidden from their patients" (p. 276).

Extrapolating the good mother ideal to the "good enough" analyst often seems to make the assumption that we are equally invested in our adult patients—not to mention the inference that they come to us in a similar *tablula rasa* state as do infants. Beebe and Lachmann (2020) have, in recent years, attempted to augment their mother-infant research and work at clarifying how the treatment relationship between adults is both similar and very different.

In addition to emphasizing that both parties come to treatment with what they call self-processes or "self-contingencies," they recently noted another critical difference between the mother/infant and analyst/patient dyads. Incorporating the research of Holtz (2004), they unsurprisingly say, "… mothers are more responsive to infants than infants are to mothers" (p. 321). It had been assumed for some time that analysts are responsive to their patients in the same way that mothers are to infants. However, Beebe and Lachman report that Holtz's study revealed the opposite. Much to their surprise, they note, "*In contrast, patients are more responsive to therapists than therapists are to patients*" (p. 321, emphasis added).

This research was very limited, and Beebe and Lachmann await further studies to see if this surprising result is replicated. I think it is likely to be replicated in further research, simply because analysts are adults who are naturally self-interested, and who have preferences, wishes, and desires that their patients become aware of, as I stated earlier. We do not seriously consider that our patients are monitoring us in the same manner that we are monitoring them, and they know where the power lies in the relationship. To some extent, they know they need to satisfy us to get what they need.

Patients, of course, want to influence the analyst as well, but are not on equal footing in terms of personal power in the relationship. Holtz's research suggests a power differential that we all know is there, but we are reluctant to acknowledge in an era that eschews analytic authority and power, emphasizing co-construction and mutual influence instead. But as Aron (1996) said, mutuality and symmetry are not the same thing. In the end, the power—and, as per Mitchell (1998), the *responsibility*—lie with the analyst.

The threat posed by negative feelings

Like most of us, Mitchell seemed most comfortable when he was empathically in tune with his patients and feeling positively toward them. In fact, a case example of his negative feelings toward a patient is oft-quoted, both for his candor and the difficulty in locating a suitable approach to expressing frustration and anger toward a patient. How does one do this while still maintaining the therapeutic relationship?

Mitchell (2000) reports on the case of Helen, a patient who he could not satisfy. In response to her criticisms, he reported fluctuating between excessive informality and excessive formality. On this latter point, he describes himself as "acting formally and pretending to be warm." The pretense of warmth was, of course, the best he could muster in the midst of her scathing criticism of him—illustrating that we cannot escape our normal and expectable reactions as human beings. Mitchell's subsequent interactions with her point to the fact that not only can we not hide our true feelings—our patients do not want us to try. Mitchell describes their interaction as follows:

I tried in different ways to describe her conflicts concerning how she wanted me to be, but that just made her angrier. After about half hour of these attacks, she turned up the heat. "How come I can't get a human response out of you?" She taunted. "I know you are hating me. Why don't you just come out and say it. Look, if we were out on the street, if this weren't an analytic relationship. What would you say to me right now?"

I felt trapped. Given the increasing anger I was feeling, it seemed that either salience or an interpretation would be provocative, yet I couldn't think of anything to say that wouldn't be simply retaliatory. I ended up saying something like, "If this were *not* an analytic relationship, if we were out on the street and you were talking to me this way and I weren't your analyst, I probably would say 'FUCK YOU.' But I am your analyst."

She laughed, and I laughed, and the tension was broken. (p. 142)

Mitchell says Helen risked confronting him and even offered a kind of transitional space that allowed him to express himself constructively. He said he was able to express his negative feelings while emphasizing his position and responsibilities as her analyst.

I have no doubt that many clinicians would regard this as an enactment, yet consider that Mitchell's feelings were far from unconscious. He was feeling intensely but unsure how to proceed in a manner that would be therapeutic. As he rightly says, Helen not only brought his feelings into the room but also practically gave him his lines. I continue to be impressed with the frequency with which even the most difficult patients will provide the same type of instructions that Helen provided for Mitchell. Yet we cannot count on that. Many patients are far too afraid of acknowledging mutual anger or rage, fearing destruction of either one of the participants and/or the relationship.

I like to think that Steve Mitchell would be open to looking at this example as both a conflict that was resolved through an affective exchange and as one illustrating that the analyst's frustration, anger, and other negative affects can be successfully verbalized.

Perhaps more importantly, his example illustrates the type of stalemate that inevitably occurs when feelings are denied or suppressed. Perhaps our deep reluctance to express anger toward patients could be overcome more easily if we could admit to our fears of doing harm, as stated previously. I think the case of Helen demonstrates how often our patients are seeking our emotional honesty rather than our protection.

I state repeatedly in this volume that I believe we have over-emphasized the role of enactment because it fits so well with the passivity of the analysts and our need to see ourselves as always good and well-intentioned. At the heart of many discussions of enactment is the analyst's and patient's mutual helplessness—their inability to know what they are feeling or to express it. This belief virtually eliminates the analyst's responsibility to bring conflict to light. If analysts truly cannot not know their feelings prior to enactment, as Levenson (1996) and Renik (1993) propose, what is the point of analytic treatment? Is it not self-awareness? Does it no longer offer the prospect of bringing unconscious thoughts and feelings into awareness? If it does, then why do some analysts embrace a lack of awareness?

The enactment perspective implies that constructive conflict cannot be cultivated. Rather, it remains as an inevitable tsunami, uprooting the dyad until they regain control and attempt to sort out what has just happened. In this new paradigm shift, both analyst and patient are essentially innocent. They do not wish each other ill. They are the victims of their own early attachments and traumatic experiences, not matter how badly they behave.

In line with this paradigm shift, negative feelings toward patients are increasingly viewed as necessarily fleeting, uncommon, and potentially a sign of an analyst who is lacking in sufficient empathy and compassion. A "good" analyst is one who can perform a holding function indefinitely and who primarily experiences and expresses negative feelings toward patients while in the throes of an enactment. By definition, the enactment of negative countertransference is seen as unintentional and anomalous. More recently, Mark (2018), in speaking of our reliance on enactment, says,

> In this charged atmosphere in which bad-me states are so difficult
> to inhibit, a multi-faceted spiraling process is initiated, in which the

analyst's experiential freedom narrows. The analyst tries harder and harder to be "understanding" and "helpful." Increasingly, there becomes only room for the analyst's good-me. (p. 82)

Managing negative feelings and conflict

This resistance to knowing our negative thoughts and feelings is a barrier to needed self-awareness. Modell (1991), writing as the emphasis on the inevitability of ongoing countertransference was being integrated into analytic thought, noted that analysts are relieved when they discover that their negative feelings toward a patient are part in response to a clearly defined transference. However, when this is not the case,

> we are uneasy when our negative reactions, such as our dislike of a patient, cannot be woven into the fabric of the treatment process, for this situation is a threat to our professional persona and a threat to our work ego. (pp. 21–22)

The cumulative psychotherapy research, rarely cited in the psychoanalytic literature, confirms that the therapist's unresolved conflicts and resulting negative feelings toward patients result in unsuccessful treatments when they are acted out rather than managed. Management may include deliberate disclosure but does not include enactment, and therapists who were keenly aware of negative feelings actually had more successful outcomes than therapists who were not (Hayes & Nelson, 2015).

As Modell (1991) points out, we are reluctant to admit to negative feelings toward our patients and the ongoing unresolved conflicts that often generate them. Safran and Muran (2002), whose work is often used as a justification for quickly ending conflict within the analytic relationship, are less often quoted for their concern about *conflict avoidance* in treatment, bemoaning the lack of discussion about dealing with the analyst's internal struggles in treatment.

I have long advocated for the necessity of an asymmetrical but mutual emotional surrender in treatment. However, this is not an easy achievement. It requires not only a high degree of self-awareness and more than a little ego strength, but also a commitment to accepting both our patients' and our own limitations. It requires an appreciation for the mutual desire to influence each other that begins with the first session. Both analyst and patient must have in place a system of defenses that serve to maintain their own intrapsychic equilibrium. Yet the analyst would ideally be capable of leading the way toward working through conflicts that create too much emotional isolation.

Conflict and the aggression that ensues are a natural consequence of having our own emotional territory, for lack of a better word. I think we often ignore the fact that one of the main functions of affect is to influence and that both analyst and patient seek constantly to influence each other and naturally wish to dominate. Solms (2020) talks about the 60-40 rule in relationships, noting that who is on which end can fluctuate, but that when this basic balance is disturbed, the relationship does not work. Insufficient attention to this inherent power struggle, in the interests of maintaining the analyst's persona as non-power-seeking and benevolent, denies both members of the dyad access to a basic reality. Hirsch (1997) frankly describes the scenario that often unfolds with patients who resist being influenced:

> The analyst's sadism can readily be expressed by a view of the patient as a deficient, weak, egoless or arrested as a child. The analyst defends against impotent rage by treating the patient as if he or she is a helpless, pitiable child and by acting with a cloying kindness which is not at all genuinely experienced. (pp. 252–253)

Searles (1966) was the first person to directly address the issue of how analysts can deal with negative responses to patients, both intrapsychically and interpersonally. He offered examples with his own patients, as Hirsch has pointed out. But much of his clinical work was not considered applicable to outpatient psychoanalytic because he worked with borderline and schizophrenic inpatients. Bird (1972) notes that at times we defensively respond too quickly to the patient's anger: "When angry accusations do come from the patient, we nip them off too prematurely and may even couch our interpretations in just the right way to clear ourselves of the accusations" (p. 289).

McLaughlin (1987), another pioneer in humanizing the analytic process, described his own reaction formation in response to an angry patient: "Meanwhile I had grown aware that I was being spooked into excessive helpfulness by my anger and need to deny it" (p. 571). Gabbard (1995) has also repeatedly emphasized that confronting our negative feelings toward patients has been arguably our greatest weakness and the cause of passive submission. He notes that pacifying angry patients is not only untherapeutic but also leads to all manner of boundary violations, ranging from excessive concessions to sexual misconduct.

Reviewing this literature on negative countertransference, created before the formal Relational movement had even begun, I am inspired anew by the brilliance and humility of these authors. At the same time, I am a bit saddened to realize that we have never taken up the call to address these difficult issues in any consistent, strategic way. Most important, of course, would be some discourse about what seems to be effective ways of dealing with countertransference anger. I agree with Ormont (1992), who speaks of the challenge of expressing "creative rage."

If we could gather more information on what people actually do in treatment, we might be able to distill our clinical wisdom into something teachable. Unfortunately, perhaps intrinsic to the denial that arises when we feel anger or rage toward a patient, intellectual and emotional examinations escape us. We are also equally as prone to defending ourselves when attacked as anyone else. I do not note this as a fault, but rather a human trait that we are compelled to process more constructively as part of our responsibility to our patients.

The flip side of dealing with anger toward our aggressive patients, of course, is the aforementioned overly peaceful relationship, untainted by anger on either side of the dyad. Safran et al. (2014) reveal their research shows that patients report having had negative feelings towards their therapists that the therapists were completely unaware of. I think this says something about our need to dispatch any anger, and the potential for conflict, out of awareness. Our individual aversion to conflict naturally creates a therapeutic culture that discourages the revelation of negative emotions and thoughts about patients. Mills (2004) is characteristically frank on this topic.

The admission of extreme negative feelings about a patient is typically met with a consternation if not moral reproach for being so brazen (and remiss) in offering such a candid confession. As a result, students and clinicians alike are discouraged from discussing their true feelings in professional space…due to a culture of dishonesty and fear that is promulgated from within the academy and analytic institutes regarding standards of training and professional identity. (p. 482)

In speaking to both experienced analysts and those in training, it becomes clear that expectable negative feelings, including triggering the analyst's unresolved conflicts, is not adequately addressed in analytic training. I believe Mills is correct about not only the neglect of negative countertransference, but the institutionalized shame that keeps it suppressed. Confronting these topics directly in training is essential to adequately preparing new analysts to deal with the onslaught of intense feelings that awaits them in analytic work.

Conclusion

Contrary to popular opinion, Relational theory was infused with the importance of conflict in the early writings of Stephen Mitchell (1988). Yet the subject of interpersonal conflict has never taken hold in the two-person approach. Rather, it has become subsumed under the rubric of enactment.

This chapter has focused on our early experiences as family caregivers as a partial explanation for the tendency for analysts being conflict avoidant. Research on early attachments and the need for holding and empathy have prevailed as a model for clinical interventions, creating a parentified and overly passive approach to doing treatment. Additionally, the persona of the analyst has increasingly centered on self-sacrifice rather than authenticity. Along with this revised view of the analyst has come a neglect of both conflict and negative countertransference, privileging the role of the good mother. It is my belief that an empathic, caring, and responsible approach to treatment need not exclude a recognition of mutual influence and the inevitability of conflict.

References

Aron, L. (1991). The patient's experience of the analyst's subjectivity. *Psychoanalytic Dialogues*, *1*, 29–51.

Aron, L. (1996). *A meeting of minds: Mutuality in context*. Hillsdale, NJ: The Analytic Press.

Beebe, B., & Lachmann, F. (2020). Infant research and adult treatment revisited: Cocreating self- and interactive regulation. *Psychoanalytic Psychology*, *37*, 313–323.

Bird, B. (1972). Notes on transference: Universal phenomenon and hardest part of analysis. *Journal of the American Psychoanalytic Association*, *20*, 267–301.

Bowlby, J. (1969). *Attachment and loss, Vol. 1: Attachment*. New York: Basic Books.

Bowlby, J. (1973). *Attachment and loss, Vol. 2: Separation*. New York: Basic Books.

Brenner, C. (2008). Aspects of psychoanalytic theory: Drives, defense, and the pleasure-unpleasure principle. *Psychoanalytic Quarterly*, *77*, 707–717.

Busch, F. (2005). Conflict theory/Trauma theory. *Psychoanalytic Quarterly*, *74*, 27–45.

Celenza, A. (2007). Analytic love and power: Responsiveness and responsibility. *Psychoanalytic Inquiry*, *27*, 287–301.

Celenza, A. (2010). The analyst's need and desire. *Psychoanalytic Dialogues*, *20*, 60–69.

Christian, C. (2015). Intersubjectivity and modern conflict theory. *Psychoanalytic Psychology*, *32*, 608–622.

Dent, L., & Christian, C. (2019). The shifting prevalence of conflict in psychoanalytic literature: A brief report of a corpus-based text analysis. *Psychoanalytic Psychology*, *36*, 184–188.

Dunbar, N. E. (2015). A review of theoretical approaches to interpersonal power. *Review of Communication*, *15*, 1–18.

Erikson, E. H. (1950). *Childhood and society*. New York: Norton.

Fairbairn, W. R. D. (1954). *An object-relations theory of the personality*. New York: Basic Books.

Gabbard, G. (1995). *Boundaries and boundary violations in psychoanalysis*. New York: Basic Books.

Gabbard, G. (1997). A reconsideration of objectivity in the analyst. *International Journal of Psychoanalysis*, *78*, 15–26.

Guntrip, H. (1969). *Schizoid phenomena, object relations and the self*. New York: International Universities Press.

Harris, A. (2005). Conflict in relational treatments. *Psychoanalytic Quarterly, 74*, 267–293.

Hayes, J. A., Nelson, D. L. B., & Fauth, J. (2015). Countertransference in successful and unsuccessful cases of psychotherapy. *Psychotherapy, 52*, 127–133.

Hirsch, I. (1987). Varying modes of analytic participation. *Journal of the American Academy of Psychoanalysis, 15*, 205–222.

Hirsch, I. (1997). Analytic intimacy, analyzability and the vulnerable analyst. *Free Association, 7*, 250–259.

Holtz, P. (2004). The self-and interactive regulation and coordination of vocal rhythms, interpretive accuracy, and progress in brief psychodynamic psychotherapy. *Dissertation Abstracts International: B, The Sciences and Engineering, 64m* 3526.

Kohut, H. (1971). *The analysis of the self.* New York: International Universities Press.

LeDoux, J. (1994). Memory versus emotional memory in the brain. In P. Eckman & R. Davidson (Eds.), *The nature of emotion: Fundamental questions* (pp. 311–312). New York: Oxford University Press.

Levenson, E. A. (1996). Aspects of self-revelation and self-disclosure. *Contemporary Psychoanalysis, 32*, 237–248.

Mahler, M., Pine, F., & Bergman, A. (1975). *The psychological birth of the human infant: Symbiosis and individuation.* New York: Basic Books.

Mark, D. (2018). Forms of equality in relational analysis. In L. Aron, S. Grand, & J. Slochower (Eds.), *De-idealizing relational theory: A critique from within* (pp. 80-101). London: Routledge.

Maroda, K. (1991). *The power of countertransference: innovations in analytic technique.* Chichester, UK: Wiley.

Maroda, K. (2004). A relational perspective on women and power. *Psychoanalytic Psychology, 21*, 428–435.

McLaughlin, J. (1987). The play of transference: Some reflections on enactment in the psychoanalytic situation. *Journal of the American Psychoanalytic Association, 35*, 557–582.

Mills, J. (2004). Countertransference revisited. *Psychoanalytic Review, 91*, 467–515.

Mitchell, S. A. (1984). Object relations theories and the developmental tilt. *Contemporary Psychoanalysis, 20*, 473–499.

Mitchell, S. A. (1988). *Relational concepts in psychoanalysis: An integration.* Cambridge, MA: Harvard University Press.

Mitchell, S. A. (1998). *Influence and autonomy in psychoanalysis.* Hillsdale, NJ: The Analytic Press.

Mitchell, S. A. (2000). *Relationality: From attachment to intersubjectivity.* Hillsdale, NJ: The Analytic Press.

Modell, A. H. (1991). The therapeutic relationship as a paradoxical experience. *Psychoanalytic Dialogues, 1,* 13–28.

Nunberg, H. (1934). The feeling of guilt. *Psychoanalytic Quarterly, 3:* 589–604.

Ormont, L. R. (1992). Subjective countertransference in the group setting: The modern analytic experience. *Modern Psychoanalysis, 17,* 3–12.

Renik, O. (1993). Analytic interactions: Conceptualizing technique in light of the analyst's irreducible subjectivity. *Psychoanalytic Quarterly, 62,* 553–571.

Safran, J. D., Muran, J. C., & Shaker, A. (2014). Research on therapeutic impasses and ruptures in the therapeutic alliance. *Contemporary Psychoanalysis, 50,* 211–232.

Safran, J., & Muran, J. C. (2002). *Negotiating the therapeutic alliance.* New York: Guilford.

Schore, A. N. (1994). *Affect regulation and the origin of the self: The neurobiology of emotional development.* Hillsdale, NJ: Lawrence Erlbaum Associates.

Schore, A. N. (2001a). The effects of a secure attachment relationship on right-brain development, affect regulation, and infant mental health. *Infant Mental Health Journal, 22,* 7–66.

Schore, A. N. (2001b). The seventh Annual John Bowlby Memorial Lecture. Minds in the making: Attachment, the self-organizing brain, and developmentally-oriented psychoanalytic psychotherapy. *British Journal of Psychotherapy, 17,* 299–328.

Searles, H. (1966). Feelings of guilt in the psychoanalyst. *Psychiatry, 29,* 319–323.

Slavin, M. O., & Kriegman, D. K. (1998). Why the analyst needs to change: Toward a theory of conflict. *Psychoanalytic Dialogues, 8,* 247–284.

Slochower, J. (2018). Going too far: Relational heroines and relational excess. In L. Aron, S. Grand, & J. Slochower (Eds.), *De-idealizing relational theory: A critique from within* (pp. 8–34). London: Routledge.

Solms, M. (2020). *Mark Solms teaches from lockdown.* Retrieved from https://mark-solms-in-lock-down.teachable.com/courses/enrolled/860398

Sperry, M. (2011). This better be good! Complex systems and the dread of influence. *International Journal of Psychoanalytic Psychology, 6,* 74–98.

Stern, D. (1985). *The interpersonal world of the infant.* New York: Basic Books.

Wachtel, P. (2017). The relationality of everyday life: The unfinished journey of relational psychoanalysis. *Psychoanalytic Dialogues, 27,* 503–521.

Welt, S. R., & Herron, W. G. (1990). *Narcissism and the psychotherapist.* New York: Guilford.

Wilson, M. (2013). Desire and responsibility: The ethics of counter-transference experience. *The Psychoanalytic Quarterly, 82,* 435–476.

Winnicott, D. W. (1960). The theory of the parent-infant relationship. *International Journal of Psychoanalysis, 41,* 585–595.

Wolf, A. W., Goldfried, M. R., & Muran, J. C. (2017). Therapist negative reactions: How to transform toxic experiences. In L. G. Castonguay & C. E. Hill (Eds.), *How and why are some therapists better than others? Understanding therapist effects* (pp. 175-192). Washington, DC: American Psychological Association.

Chapter 5

Deconstructing enactment

One of the most fascinating and perplexing expressions of uncon-scious-to-unconscious communication is enactment. Having been accepted as inevitable,[1] the actual clinical management of enact-ment remains vague. Understanding the role of consciousness and also the therapeutic action of self-disclosure are essential to a rea-sonable definition of enactment. However, current use of the term *unconscious* is arguably dated and misapplied in discussions of im-plicit, ongoing communication.

Virtually all examples in the literature of processed enactments contain two elements: The first is a discussion of what emotions in both analyst and patient were out of awareness at the time of the enactment; the second is what type of disclosure was needed to adequately process the analyst's participation. Clinicians typically state that they assess the patient's need for disclosure post-enactment, emphasizing that this can only be done in the present moment. As a result, the lack of guidelines for self-disclosure leaves clinicians in training with little guidance in this area. We ac-knowledge that self-disclosure is often needed, and works, without having any formal theory for its therapeutic action vis-á-vis en-actment. Presenters and authors often go much further, warning against attempting to establish any guidelines for technique, as Busch (2003) has pointed out.

The evolving definition of enactment

To set the context for this discussion, we first need to examine the varying uses and definitions of enactment. Bohleber et al. (2013) highlight the rapidly evolving nature of the term *enactment*, yet set their sights on delineating the universal characteristics that cut across the multiple existing definitions.

> Suddenly, something seems to be incomplete; the analyst is thrown off balance, he loses the sense of his normal analytic functioning, and this sudden awareness of discontinuity causes a disruption in the phenomenological field … the process is described by the various authors in a fairly similar way: "The analyst does … get emotionally involved … in a manner he had not intended" (Boesky, 1990, p. 573). Every description indicates the existence of a certain pressure to act on the part of the analyst, which at the time he does not understand. One might say that the analyst "catches himself in the act." (p. 510)

I (Maroda, 1998) described these universal qualities, while also emphasizing the mutuality and emotional vulnerability inherent in enactment.

> Enactment is an affectively driven repetition of converging emotional scenarios from the patient's and the analyst's lives. It is not merely an affectively driven set of behaviors; it is necessarily a repetition of past events that have been buried in the unconscious due to associated unmanageable or unwanted emotion. (p. 119)

I think both of these definitions capture the essence of enactment, focusing on the unacceptability of certain feelings for both analyst and patient that are dispatched to unconscious processes. Each can be said to be experiencing some ego-dystonic emotional response that must be split off and/or projected onto the other. Interestingly, Bohleber et al. (2013) also note that enactment is a "phenomenon concerned with actions. What is missing in psychoanalysis is a comprehensive theory of action" (p. 525). So, enactment is an action that mysteriously takes place through unconscious processes that we do not really have an adequate theoretical framework to understand—even after the fact.

Prior to Jacobs' coining of the term *enactment* in 1986, this mutual unconscious event was often referred to as expressed mutual projective identification followed by mutual acting out. Jacobs (2018) says the term *enactment* just came to him because he was seeking to find a term that did not have the pejorative connotations of "acting out." He wanted to encourage clinicians to explore this phenomenon with an open mind.

The definition of enactment as an affect-driven unconscious-to-unconscious event that takes both parties by surprise, with the analyst sometimes feeling out of control, has now been labeled as a "discrete" enactment. Moreover, discussions of mutual projective identification as the precursor to action have become less frequent. Straying further from Jacobs' original definition, enactment is becoming increasingly used to describe the ongoing dynamics in the analytic dyad, as well as the miscellaneous countertransference emotions and events that take the analyst by surprise. Gabbard (1995) reminds us that, by definition, enactment requires action, not just mutual affect.

In an attempt to clarify our use of enactment, Bass (2003) has proposed that the ongoing unconscious engagement be called enactment with a little "e" and discrete, more powerful events that come into awareness be called enactment with a big "E." His conceptualization helps acknowledge different types of unconscious to unconscious communication in the analytic relationships. Yet, this redefining of the term *enactment* is not without controversy, as Aron (2003) observes:

> The clash is between defining enactment narrowly so that it maintains specific meaning and is thought to represent only episodic, discrete events, or define it so broadly as to alert us to the ubiquity of unconscious interpersonal mutual influence and in so doing turning all of analysis into one huge enactment. (p. 622)

I also believe that we tend to over apply many concepts in psychoanalysis once they become popular. This certainly happened with the term *empathy*, particularly in the heyday of self-psychology. I personally believe that it is important to name the phenomenon we observe and to have an agreed-upon working definition that can help expand our thinking, both theoretically and clinically. I agree with Aron that once a term has been overapplied in both narrow and broad terms, it loses meaning. Why not take the concept of ongoing communication, at all levels of consciousness, and simply refer to it as such? The term *enactment* can then be used to refer to a particular and distinctive subset of that communication, as originally intended. For my purposes, I will limit my use of the term *enactment* to refer to the discrete, observable event that is affect-driven, characterized by a lack of awareness and frequently discombobulating. (See Ivey, 2008, for a detailed discussion of theoretical debates regarding the nature of enactment.)

Self-disclosure

The next term that requires some definition is *self-disclosure*, particularly as it is used in discussions of enactment. Renik (1997), Levenson (1996), and others have strongly asserted that countertransference affect cannot be fully known and experienced until after it has emerged through enactment. Levenson (1996) was the first to take this position: "Really troublesome countertransference operates well out of awareness. It usually takes some acting-out (on either side) or a dream (again, on either side) to be exposed" (p. 240). I think these views have helped to endorse the clinical usefulness and desirability of enactment, seeing it as bringing to light that which otherwise would have laid dormant in the unconscious. Subsequently, self-disclosure becomes permissible, if not inevitable, for the purposes of adequately processing an enactment. Once the analyst's feelings have surfaced, some admission and explanation generally take place. It is hard to deny that after an angry outburst toward the patient, for example, a conversation about the analyst's anger would naturally ensue.

It should be noted that case examples in the literature illustrating this process are often followed by warnings about not self-disclosing as a matter of course. The authors typically emphasize the uniqueness of every analytic dyad and the impossibility of predicting what will be needed regarding self-disclosure, if anything at all. The end result is that we continue to share clinical experiences without linking our behaviors (e.g., our self-disclosures) with any underlying principle that might be applied more generally. (This point illustrates the earlier quote from Bohleber et al., 2013, regarding our lack of a theoretical framework for understanding what is actually happening in an enactment.) And Wachtel (2008) has said, "The essence of the relational view on self-disclosure is not that one is *required* to self-disclose but that one is *permitted* to. The differences and implications for clinical practice of these two understandings is very considerable" (p. 245).

Requiring self-disclosure would not sit well with most analytic clinicians, of course. But the repeated conversations about enactment clearly demonstrate the ubiquity of self-disclosure in post-enactment conversations. Ivey (2008) also makes the argument that self-disclosure is an inevitable critical element, albeit unintended, in the enactment process. But, in line with the widespread confusion and ambivalence about deliberate disclosure, he asks:

> [I]s further *intentional* self-disclosure concerning our involvement in and experience of the interactions appropriate? If so, what form of disclosure might optimally facilitate the exploration and resolution of the specific enactment dynamic without disturbing the analytic relationship and emotionally burdening the patient with details of our own psychic conflicts? (p. 33)

Ivey is not alone in the fear that deliberate disclosure will do harm to the patient. But has our fear of doing harm prevented us from responsibly exploring the therapeutic value of self-disclosure and its appropriate uses? I think this is yet another instance when the underlying fears of the analyst, rooted in early childhood experience, dominate our clinical choices.

One source of the debate on self-disclosure revolves around *what* material is disclosed. Levenkron (2006) describes an enactment where she struggles with whether or not to tell her patient that their relationship is fraying, in part, because they are both going through a divorce. She ultimately decides not to share this personal information. Rather, she processes her immediate anger after it erupts in relation to the patient. She intuitively realizes that it is her emotional response to the patient that is most important, rather than the details of her personal life. I often find that patients feel burdened by personal information unless it is absolutely needed to explain the analyst's emotional state. (While these may vary and are necessarily judgment calls, certainly there is a precedent for disclosing events that involve absences, such as treatment for medical problems and illness or death in the family.)

I have frequently referred to my countertransference responses emanating from being dominated by an older sister, yet notice that my patients rarely ask any for any details about this at all. I simply tell them that someone early in my life was often angry and controlling and that I sometimes overreact when someone treats me this way in the present. I can't recall a time when any patient ever asked for details about this. If you accept that enactment is essentially an affective event, it makes sense that personal information potentially muddies the waters rather than providing clarity.

Perhaps another source of reluctance to formalize affective self-disclosure relates to the work that needs to be done regarding repetitive affective patterns. The current strong emphasis on the uniqueness of every analytic dyad, though indisputable to a degree, inevitably de-emphasizes the repetitive patterns in both analyst and patient that are equally inevitable. Ormont (1992) stressed therapist self-awareness of his or her countertransference, particularly the patterns that we tend to repeat over time, as essential to a positive therapeutic outcome. Certainly, all analytic clinicians are well aware of this phenomenon, and group therapists in particular do focus heavily on repetitive patterns of feeling in both therapist and patient, yet there is very little emphasis on this in the analytic literature.

The end result is both a lack of clarity in theoretical conceptualization of enactment and a lack of clarity in clinical processing. Certainly, one of the obstacles to writing about countertransference disclosure is that it necessitates some mention of the analyst's repetitive patterns and even character flaws. Clinicians are understandably reluctant to do this. Yet how can we discuss enactment productively without including at least some of this material? In reading a large number of case reports, it appears that many of them ultimately focus on the patient: For example, the patient was repeating a deadening sense of hopelessness, and the analyst naturally fell into sharing that emotional state. This falls far short of describing a mutually created event.

As stated, therapist self-disclosure invariably becomes part of the dialogue between analyst and patient, but it is only endorsed as a tool for after-the-enactment processing. Suppressed conflicts surge to the surface, ready to be addressed. And, after all, is it not one goal of analysis to make past conflicts alive in the present? And doesn't enactment further this goal? Perhaps one could even say that the working through of enactment has become the new model for therapeutic action (Aron & Atlas, 2015, Boston Change Process Study Group, 2013). The problem with relying on enactment for this purpose is that it is both unnecessarily chaotic and that *it removes both the power and the responsibility of the analyst for facilitating and processing affect in the treatment.* We tend to accept that we have no potential to control feelings that are suppressed and burst into awareness during enactment, a notion largely built on conclusions that, strictly speaking, are the opinions of the authors rather than established fact. I realize that this is inherently true of almost all clinical discussions (including this one), yet the references to the research on unconscious communication can create the appearance of an evidence-based argument for uses of enactment where none exists.

Furthermore, in reviewing case reports of enactment, it is difficult to find one where the analyst talks about his or her feelings leading up to an enactment that do not include an awareness of negative feelings toward that patient. (This is not to say that they may be temporarily unaware in the moment due the experience of objectionable and intense negative feelings.) Often, the clinician reports feeling overwhelmed, confused, and/or guilty and ashamed about the extent of his or her negative response toward the patient. *Waiting for negative countertransference feelings to pass inevitably leads to enactment.* But this is not the same as all enactments being inevitable.

Published examples of pent-up negative feelings can be found in the courageous and provocative examples of intense enactments provided by Jacobs (2001) and Chused (2003). In Jacobs' (2001) paper on enactment, he gives an example of a patient who he often found boring and "tedious." On this particular day, he was tired and fidgeting. At one point, he lost track of what the patient had been saying, which the patient detected. He had been turning the pages of his notebook and she heard it. When she said it sounded like he was fingering something, he diverted to talking about the male babysitter who had touched her inappropriately while reading to her before bedtime. Jacobs notes that after making a reference to "stroking," the patient talked freely about this event with the babysitter, basically going along with his efforts to deflect her attention away from what he had been doing. All appeared to be well during that session. But then Jacobs says,

> After that session, Ms N's distrust of me increased. Her resistances hardened and silences dominated the sessions. When she did speak, what she said was mostly reportage; dispatches consisting largely of descriptions of other people ... She had gone into hiding and the reason for this was clear. In some part of her Ms N knew that I had deceived her with a piece of psychoanalytic sleight of hand. Out of boredom, anger and a wish to escape from those feelings, I had turned away from Ms N. and tuned her out. (p. 663)

Feeling quite guilty and realizing (in his own words) that he had "gaslighted" her, he brought the subject up and apologized, which allowed them to work through this conflict and move forward.

Chused's (2003) paper on enactment demonstrates an enviable admission of failure to accept and acknowledge the countertransference as being at the heart of enactment. She gives an example of an often-critical patient who berates her for noise in an adjoining room of Chused's home office. The patient compares Chused to a personal shopper she is unhappy with and says neither of them is earning their money. Chused admits to feeling insulted and makes these defensive comments to the patient: "Yes, you are paying me to use my skill to help you, but the skill is mine, developed by me, and it is put in the service of helping you because I wish to help you" (p. 678).

The patient is silent for a while, then says Chused sounds angry, then is silent again and says she guesses that she had hurt Chused. A few sessions later, the patient is talking about how she knows her mother loves her even though she could never adequately express it. Again, there is noise, this time from an adolescent patient in the waiting room singing loudly with his headphones on. The patient again is silent, then asks Chused about the noise; Chused said it bothered her but there was nothing she could do about it. The patient simply says, "But you could have told him to be quiet." Chused does not hesitate to note her own motivations.

It was clear she was right. As she spoke, I realized that my inaction had been due to my feeling torn between wanting to protect her hour and not wanting to engage in a sadomasochistic exchange with the provocative teenager in the waiting room, who, in my reluctance to silence him, had continued to sing loudly. I had rationalized that to leave my patient and go to the waiting room would have hurt her by leaving her alone, so I had done nothing ... In this hour my inaction was, consciously, a result of my doing what I thought was the best compromise between two patients' needs, but unconsciously, doing what was most comfortable for me (p. 681).

Chused is frank in her admission of self-interest and conflict avoidance (and, perhaps, avoidance of the patient's feelings of love for her). I admire her self-examination, particularly with regard to the inevitable pursuit of self-interest by the analyst. I think acknowledging that we all pursue our own interests to varying degrees and in various forms helps pave the way for reducing guilt and shame, without removing responsibility for our actions.

Both of these examples illustrate both how the analyst can be aware of negative feelings toward the patient for some time, sit on those feelings, and then be confronted with an enactment that requires self-disclosure and vulnerability. I think both examples illustrate the difficulty in navigating enactments given that the analyst's defensiveness is naturally stimulated—both by the patient's responses and by internal guilt and shame.

Consciousness and enactment

A second questionable assumption regarding enactment involves the question of consciousness. What does unconscious-to-unconscious communication really mean, particularly from session to session, or moment to moment? Studies on levels of consciousness (Berlin, 2012, Hassein et al., 2005) point to a continuum where conscious control varies constantly, depending on the person's need for vigilance, with the assumed goal of physical and psychic survival. Yet if most of what we do is decided in the unconscious, what hope is there for the efficacy of any conscious-to-conscious communication as the basis for change, be it psychotherapy or psychoanalysis? Is the Boston Change Process Study Group correct in their assumption that psychoanalytic treatment is essentially a *right brain to right brain affective series of events that can only be minimally facilitated at the conscious level?* And, that unconscious material surfaces primarily as the result of an enactment?

Before much of the current work in neuropsychology, people equated unconscious control *with no control.* On the contrary, behaviors of all sorts, including self-disclosure, that appear to be spontaneous and uncontrolled are actually controlled by a system of internalized knowledge, values, experience, and emotional reactions that are primarily out of awareness. As Hassein et al. (2005) says in *The New Unconscious*, "Non-conscious control is not only logically possible, it is a psychological reality" (p. 215). In the same edited volume, Glaser & Kihlstrom (2005) note that "the human mind is capable of maintaining unconscious control over its own automatic processes. This suggests a volitional nature of the unconscious, an idea that too many may seem self-contradictory" (p. 189).

What is learned becomes automatic. Even painfully self-conscious actions are eventually mastered and controlled by unconscious processes. It seems ironic to me that a bedrock of psychoanalytic thought, developing the awareness of unconscious feelings, values, and intentions, is currently being undermined by those who believe that unconscious communication should be our primary focus. Ginot (2015) says,

> In spite of the emphasis on therapeutic enactments, these models do not sufficiently stress the ongoing reciprocal exchange between the two realms (Damasio, 2010; Schore, 2012). Unconscious processes are not separate from conscious ones: there is a dynamic relationship between the realms affecting and influencing each other. (p. xvii)

Making a complex subject even more complex, it seems that we need to integrate the notion of an ever-changing level of conscious awareness with the idea that even unconscious processes are controlled in that they reflect the values, ideas, and feelings of the individual. Reducing the complex nature of consciousness to a binary or even trinary notion of consciousness is simply not congruent with the current research. Furthermore, it limits our ability to conceptualize our own varying emotional responses, especially over time. What is conscious at one moment can be thoroughly out of awareness at another.

Use of self-disclosure

We do not have a working definition of therapeutic self-disclosure. Even though enactment focuses on repressed affect, analyst self-disclosure is not limited to affect and, in many case reports, the analyst's feelings are minimized or avoided out of fear of harming a vulnerable patient. So what is important for the analyst to reveal—affect, personal information, both? Moreover, we do not appear to be seeking a model for therapeutic self-disclosure out of the belief that no general principles exist and that any guidelines will become prescriptive and nonresponsive to the demands of a unique dyad. (I outline my own theory of the therapeutic action of self-disclosure in Maroda, 2010.)

Incorporating some of my previous points, we do not seriously consider that while we cannot avoid all enactments, we could effectively minimize them through self-awareness and deliberate disclosure of countertransference emotion. I make this point not because I have discarded the potential benefits of enactment. Certainly, they exist. Nor do I lack the understanding that patients who have little access to their feelings frequently instigate enactment because it is simply the only way for them to express themselves. Rather, I am responding to what I believe has become an over-reliance on enactment for tapping into primitive feelings.

A close read of case examples of enactment reveal that the analyst was well aware of burgeoning negative feelings toward the patient, and the treatment, prior to enactment. And it was the suppression of these emotions that led to the enactment. The problem addressed here is one that has confounded analysts for decades: How do we harness negative countertransference emotions in the interests of furthering the treatment? There is no simple answer to this question. But I believe that we have not focused enough on identifying the analyst's negative feelings and working toward a model for constructive disclosure. Perhaps this is because of the guilt and shame associated with these feelings, and the fact that is at odds with our persona of "good enough mother."

I find it useful to think about what is occurring prior to enactment. What are the conditions that set the stage for enactment? First, and foremost, of course, is the analyst's persistent negative emotions. Often these emotions are shared.

In working toward what precedes an enactment, it seems to me that as negative feelings toward the patient, or in response to sharing the patient's affective state, are repeated over time, a gradual emotional withdrawal occurs. The analyst may be aware of not wanting to see the patient, falling into feelings of helplessness, feeling thwarted when interventions do not produce the desired results. From my clinical experience, and in reading the case reports of others, *disengagement* typically precedes enactment. It is defensive, seeking to avoid threatening stimuli from the patient and internal conflicts over guilt and shame (a point made by Chused, 2003). It is often, or perhaps always, a repetition for both analyst and patient.

If we think about enactment as expressed mutual projective identification, you may recall that the purpose of projective identification came to be seen not as a "dumping" of intolerable affect on the analyst, but rather as a way to communicate unacceptable feelings for the purpose of emotional engagement. Once we realized that projective identification was mutual, however, much of this discussion of its dynamic function faded.

In other words, enactment may well be the unconscious effort by one or both parties to re-engage after withdrawal. And I think this may be why we have increasingly embraced enactment. It succeeds in stimulating deep feeling, essentially forcing renewed emotional engagement. We can accept this positive mechanism, yet still strive to minimize enactment, for the simple reason that the outcome is not always good. Many enactments create new problems, especially if the analyst is out of control in the moment, or expresses such strong negative feelings that the patient has trouble feeling safe again. If we think of enactment as the unconscious effort to re-engage, then it is possible to think about observing disengagement, regardless of the reason, and attempting to re-engage without relying on enactment. Doing so also models affective awareness and expression for the patient. From my perspective, this requires a high degree of self-awareness, something we presumably cultivated in our own analysis, and the willingness and skill to disclose negative feelings constructively to our patients.

I think we cannot look at the current use of the term *enactment* without a closer look at its definition as well as why it holds so much appeal. Why does enactment speak to us in such a profound way? My own opinion centers on the fact that it necessarily involves an emotional encounter between analyst and patient and often comes on the heels of an emotional drought that is draining energy from the relationship. But is enactment necessary to resolve these emotional disengagements? As Ivey (2008) asks, "Do enactments always precede and provide prerequisite conditions for countertransference awareness and resolution?" (p. 19). Or, *could analyst and patient become more engaged without an enactment taking place, thereby minimizing the damage done by some enactments?* As stated previously, it appears that *deliberate emotional engagement* (rather than waiting for enactment) remains controversial.

Pitfalls of enactment

The position of enactment as inevitable at times (a position I agree with) has morphed into enactment as desirable—possibly being the only vehicle of awareness of deep emotions in both analyst and patient. Perhaps dramatic case reports illustrating the emergence of deep emotion between analyst and patient have contributed to this belief. However, even Jacobs (2002), who coined the term *enactment*, has revised his views, stating,

> While many countertransference enactments can be analyzed after the fact and turned to good use (Renik, 1993), some enactments are so disruptive and hurtful and have such an enduring effect on the patient, that, in essence, the treatment is seriously undermined. (p. 23)

Richards (1997), Chused (1997), and others have issued similar cautions regarding the destructive potential of some enactments. Chused (1997) states:

An enactment can inform us, but it can also misinform us. The very issues that led to the enactment, the unconscious conflicts in the analyst that have been stimulated, are active at the time of the enactment and will call forth defenses in the analyst, including that of inaccurate self-understanding. (p. 268)

These potentially disruptive effects of enactment, in my opinion, are often ignored. It is almost as though we believe that analysts are able to transcend the natural defensiveness and withdrawal that accompany a sudden awareness of unacceptable behavior. The complexity of working through an enactment and the emotional honesty required seem to be underplayed in the current literature.

Enactments take many forms and are often repeated until some working through occurs. The case of Michael illustrates a series of repetitive enactments that were not so dramatic as to create a rupture, but significantly affected the treatment nonetheless.

The case of Michael

Michael presented as a successful, late middle-aged software engineer, experiencing ongoing low-level depression. He attributed his malaise to increasing emotional distance from his wife of 20 years but acknowledged he has experienced some degree of depression throughout his life. His wife works as a paralegal. They have both settled into the culture of phones and computers, checking their texts and email messages obsessively throughout the evening. Yet they both admit to feeling lonely and wishing for more attention and affection from the other. (They do not have children.)

Michael portrays himself as the more remote of the two, readily admitting that his wife's complaints about his aloofness and tendency to withdraw are well-founded. He describes her as the person in charge, who basically runs everything in the household. Most tasks he completes are done so at her behest and under her direction. He says he dislikes being told what to do and nagged, yet likes that she "takes care of everything," leaving him free to do what he likes.

They are both hard workers who put in long hours. They also like to play hard, taking nice vacations, and enjoying fine food and wine.

They seem to get along best when they are on one of their trips, away from the pressures of work.

Michael speaks very highly of his wife, even when he mentions her complaints about him. He invariably states that she is absolutely right and that he needs to change. They are both psychologically sophisticated and have discussed how they recreate their childhood scenarios with each other, for better and for worse. When Michael mentions his wife's faults, he quickly notes that she is well aware of them and working on them, and that she is a good-hearted person who takes care of others. I have little reason to doubt this.

Yet over time, I found myself becoming increasingly uncomfortable when Michael would describe one of their negative encounters (he never used the word "fight" and rarely even used the word "argument"). He was more likely to say that they "bickered" a bit. He never offered up details about these disagreements but would reluctantly provide them when I asked. Soon it became clear to me that Michael was quite correct about his own passiveness and tendency to withdraw and feel bad about himself when criticized, but less aware of his own passive-aggressive behaviors. (It became evident that he often "forgot" to take care of things his wife had asked him to do, requiring her to constantly remind him.) Regarding his wife, he downplayed her negative behaviors, saying she was a bit "cranky" because she had a hard day at work. Over time, the outline of their conflicts became both broader and more detailed.

I began to realize that Michael's wife was quite critical, controlling, and was episodically aggressive to the point of being verbally abusive. Having had a mother with similar behaviors, Michael reacted as he had as a child, feeling ashamed, then confused, then withdrawing to protect himself. Coming out of his withdrawal often took several days or more, which over time contributed to the distance between him and his wife.

About six months into his treatment, I began to feel uncomfortable as Michael described, then defended, his wife's verbally abusive behavior. I asked him how he felt when she was so critical of him. He initially took exception to the word "critical" or any negative descriptor I applied to her behavior. As he defended her and pointed out his own flaws, I became more and more frustrated. Our conversations would usually just end with him withdrawing from *me*.

Each time, I vowed to remain more neutral and not be overcome by my own need to make him the victim and her the aggressor. Intellectually, I knew that he was colluding with her, so why was I getting so angry at her?

I repeatedly told myself to get a grip and keep perspective. Acting in a way that made him want to defend her and withdraw from me was anything but therapeutic. And yet, in spite of my best efforts, it continued. One day, I openly referred to her as verbally abusive, and Michael threw me a disapproving look and told me I did not understand her and how hard her childhood had been. I defensively said that I knew she had many fine qualities and that he loved her, but did he really feel that he deserved the way she treated him when her rage was stimulated? Again, nothing.

Michael and I were certainly in the throes of an intractable enactment. Knowing it was my responsibility to get us out of this, I asked myself why I continued to point out his wife's flaws, even when this intervention was clearly not helpful. I concluded that it related to my own childhood and being bullied by an older sibling. I felt that I did not deserve the treatment I endured and projected this onto Michael. I finally learned to better defend myself as I got older and wanted him to do the same. What I learned was that the only way to change someone else's verbally abusive behavior was to stand up to them and set limits. Michael was doing the opposite of that. And I wanted him to change, so that he would feel better, but also so I would feel better.

After much soul-searching, I felt I was ready to do better the next time Michael brought up the subject of marital discord. It was only then that I became more fully aware of Michael's role in our enactment. He once again described an argument he had with his wife. Unsurprisingly, he had said something she found incredibly annoying. She berated him for quite a long period of time. As he described her criticisms of him, I could see him visibly sinking down on the couch, as if collapsing under the weight of being "bad" and "feeling ashamed."

He then described another one of her excessively angry and critical responses to him. He looked hard at me, and I asked him how he felt. He said, "Oh, well, I know I can be annoying. I guess I can't blame her for being angry. I need to get better at changing so I don't annoy her so much." I said nothing. Michael looked surprised and repeated another criticism she made of him. Again, I said nothing. Michael threw me a quizzical look, noting my unusual silence. I waited, but he did not say more. He finally asked me what I was thinking.

It was then that I broached the subject of how he and I interacted regarding his encounters with his wife. I told him frankly that I thought our pattern of discussing their interactions was not helpful. I told him of my increasing awareness that my comments about her behavior were not well received by him, only making him feel guilty and obliged to defend her, then withdrawing from me. I told him that my pattern of responding had as much or more to do with me than him, and it was something I needed to stop doing. I apologized for being critical of his wife and told him outright that it was a countertransference response. I added that I had no real animosity toward his wife and accepted that she was, indeed, a good person.

He smiled immediately and said that he was very aware of our pattern and I was right—he did not like me implying anything negative about his wife—but didn't know what to say to me. We then talked further about both of our feelings during these enactment episodes, and I explained that, although he seemed unaware of it, he was communicating to me that his wife was too critical and angry at times. I said I thought that I might be expressing frustration and anger for him. He laughed at this, which I always take as a good sign. I said that there was clearly something in my background that led me to behave this way, but that I realized it was not helpful for him.

This conversation when extremely well. Michael said he thought I might be right, because his best friend had made similar remarks about his wife. We then talked about why it was so easy for him to find fault with himself, but not with his wife—or me. Following this session, we both became much more relaxed and easier with each other. The reader will no doubt not be surprised to learn that once I stopped pointing out his wife's bad behavior, *he* slowly began to note it and talk about his anger toward her. Without any suggestion or untoward action on my part, he also began to defend himself when she became unreasonable.

I think this example illustrates just how hard it can be to extract oneself from an enactment, particularly an insidious one that does create a dramatic breach that demands resolution. It also illustrates the different patterns of enactment that are possible. This was not a single, dramatic, breach-type enactment, nor was it simply the dynamic that existed between Michael and me overall. It was something that came up during a particular conversation (his wife's criticism and anger) and my internal responses to his denial of both her behavior and his feelings about that behavior. Though each enactment was discrete, there were multiple similar enactments before it was resolved, which is not uncommon. (These enactments did not continue after our heartfelt discussion about them.) The self-disclosure and subsequent processing with Michael demonstrate how a close read of the patient's reactions and our own internal discomfort can lead to a self-disclosure that breaks open the mutually constructed protective shell that has been built up.

I might add that this example could also be cited as evidence that some degree of enactment is inevitable. Michael felt better when I was empathic about this guilt and shame, when I asked questions and made good interpretations. Yet we still settled into a series of enactments that seems to have inevitable. Michael first had to trust me, then probably needed to have an emotional encounter with me as it pertained to his pattern of masochism in response to his wife's verbal abuse.

My enactments with Michael were not resolved as the result of some emotional outburst or protracted impasse, but rather through my awareness and willingness to be proactive with him. I talked openly with him about what I observed in our interactions and what I was feeling. Michael did not seek to know what motivated my behavior, but he was relieved that I took responsibility for my role in creating what happened between us. He did not need, or want, personal information about me. What he needed was my emotional honesty, about being stuck in an unhelpful pattern, some willingness to self-disclose and, of course, to take responsibility for my behavior.

Conclusion

Enactment remains a challenging concept for clinicians, not only because of the shifting definitions, but also because it is an immensely complicated subject. As demonstrated here, it is impossible to discuss enactment without also discussing countertransference, disclosure, the lack of theory and clinical guidelines, the analyst's repetitive patterns, theories of consciousness, and the analyst's defenses against negative feelings and conflict with patients.

If one accepts the premises presented here—that negative feelings toward the patient were in awareness prior to enactment; that these feelings lead to a gradual emotional disengagement; and that enactment is the natural unconscious attempt by both analyst and patient to re-engage—then it becomes plausible to focus on the analyst's negative feelings toward the patient, with an eye toward the analyst intervening deliberately to minimize enactment. Such interventions are likely to contain some self-disclosure, but are equally likely to contain the analyst's observations regarding a certain level of detachment, or discordance, inviting the patient to respond. I want to reiterate that while I believe that many enactments can be averted through greater awareness of and willingness to express the analyst's (usually) negative feelings, a measure of enactment is unavoidable.

Relational and intersubjective theory have brought the analyst as a person into the consulting room, with a level of participation that is both exhilarating and dizzying. Perhaps the challenge for the next generation is to truly overcome the remnants of our "neutrality," harnessing the power of our affective communication with the patient.

Note

1 See, for example, Aron (1991, 2003); Aron and Atlas (2015); Bass (2003); Black (2003); Bohleber et al. (2013); Boston Change Process Study Group (2013); Chused (1991, 1997, 2003); Grossmark (2012); Hirsch (1993, 1996); Ivey (2008); Jacobs (1986, 2001); Levenkron (2006); Maroda (1998); McLaughlin (1991); Mitchell (1988); Renik (1997); Richards (1997); Sandler (1976); and Stern (2004).

References

Aron, L. (1991). The patient's experience of the analyst's subjectivity. *Psychoanalytic Quarterly*, *1*, 29–51.

Aron, L. (2003). The paradoxical place of enactment in psychoanalysis: Introduction. *Psychoanalytic Dialogues*, *13*, 623–631.

Aron, L., & Atlas, G. (2015). Generative enactment: Memories from the future. *Psychoanalytic Dialogues*, *25*, 309–324.

Bass, A. (2003). "E" enactments in psychoanalysis: Another medium, another message. *Psychoanalytic Dialogues*, *13*, 657–675.

Berlin, H. A. (2012). The neural basis of the dynamic unconscious. *Neuropsychoanalysis*, *13*, 5–31.

Boesky, D. (1990). The psychoanalytic process and its components. *Psychoanalytic Quarterly*, *59*, 550–584.

Black, M. (2003). Enactment: Analytic musings on energy, language, and personal growth. *Psychoanalytic Dialogues*, *13*, 633–655.

Bohleber, W., Fonagy, P., Jimeniz, J. P., Scarfone, D.,Varvin, S., & Zysman, S. (2013). Towards a better use of psychoanalytic concepts: A model illustrated using the concept of enactment. *International Journal of Psychoanalysis*, *94*, 501–530.

Boston Change Process Study Group. (2013). Enactment and the emergence of new relational organization. *Journal of the American Psychoanalytic Association*, *61*, 727–749.

Busch, F. (2003). Back to the future. *Psychoanalytic Quarterly*, *72*, 201–215.

Cassoria, R. M. (2012). What happens before and after acute enactments? An exercise in clinical validation and the broadening of hypotheses. *International Journal of Psychoanalysis*, *93*, 53–80.

Chused, J. F. (1991). The evocative power of enactments. *Journal of the American Psychoanalytic Association*, *39*, 615–639.

Chused, J. F. (1997). Discussion of "Observing-participation, mutual enactment, and the new classical models" By Irwin Hirsch, PhD. *Contemporary Psychoanalysis*, *33*, 263–277.

Damasio, A. (2010). *Self comes to mind: Constructing the conscious brain.*New York: Pantheon.

Chused, J. F. (2003). The role of enactments. *Psychoanalytic Dialogues*, *13*, 677–687.

Gabbard, G. O. (1995). Countertransference: The emerging common ground. *International Journal of Psychoanalysis*, *76*, 475–485.

Ginot, E. (2015). *The neuropsychology of the unconscious*. New York: Norton.

Glaser, J., & Kihlstrom, J. F. (2005). Compensatory automaticity: Unconscious volition is not an oxymoron. In R. R. Hassein, J. S. Uleman, & J. A. Bargh (Eds.), *The new unconscious* (pp. 171–195). New York: Oxford.

Grossmark, R. (2012). The flow of enactive engagement. *Contemporary Psychoanalysis*, *48*, 287–300.

Hassein, R. R., Uleman, J. S. & Bargh, J. A. (Eds.) (2005). *The new unconscious*. New York: Oxford.

Hirsch, I. (1993). Countertransference enactments and some issues related to external factors in the analyst's life. *Psychoanalytic Dialogues, 3*, 343–366.

Hirsch, I. (1996). Observing-participation, mutual enactment, and the new classical models. *Contemporary Psychoanalysis, 32*, 359–383.

Ivey, G. (2008). Enactment controversies: A critical review of current debates. *International Journal of Psychoanalysis, 89*, 19–38.

Jacobs, T. J. (1986). On countertransference enactments. *Journal of the American Psychoanalytic Association, 34*, 289–307.

Jacobs, T. J. (2001). On misleading and misreading patients: Some reflections on communications, miscommunications, and countertransference enactments. *International Journal of Psychoanalysis, 82*, 653–669.

Jacobs, T. J. (2002). Secondary revision: On rethinking the analytic process and analytic technique: *Psychoanalytic Inquiry, 22*, 3–28.

Jacobs, T. J. (2018) Theodore J. Jacobs "On countertransference enactments." *PEP/UCL Top Authors Project, 1*, 25.

Levenkron, H. (2006). Love (and hate) with the proper stranger: Affective honesty and enactment. *Psychoanalytic Inquiry, 26*, 157–181.

Levenson, E. (1996). Aspects of self-revelation and self-disclosure. *Contemporary Psychoanalysis, 32*, 237–247.

Maroda, K. (2010). *Psychodynamic techniques: Working with emotion in the therapeutic relationship*. New York: Guilford.

Maroda, K. (1998). Enactment: When the patient's and analyst's pasts converge. *Psychoanalytic Psychology, 15*, 517–535.

McLaughlin, J. T. (1991). Clinical and theoretical aspects of enactment. *Journal of the American Psychoanalytic Association, 39*, 595–614.

Mitchell, S. (1988). *Relational concepts in psychoanalysis*. Cambridge, MA: Harvard University Press.

Ormont, L. (1992). Subjective countertransference in the group setting: The modern analytic experience. *Modern Psychoanalysis, 17*, 3–12.

Renik, O. (1993). Analytic interaction: Conceptualizing technique in light of the analyst's irreducible subjectivity. *Psychoanalytic Quarterly, 62*, 553–571.

Renik, O. (1997). Reactions to "Observing-participation, mutual enactment, and the new classical models, by Irwin Hirsch, PhD. *Contemporary Psychoanalysis, 33*, 279–284.

Richards, A. (1997, July). Interaction in the transference/countertransference continuum. Paper presented at the meeting of the International Psychoanalytic Association, Barcelona, Spain.

Sandler, J. (1976). Countertransference and role-responsiveness. *International Review of Psychoanalysis, 3,* 43–47.

Schore, A. N. (2012). *The science of the art of psychotherapy.* New York: Norton.

Stern, D. B. (2004). The eye sees itself: Dissociation, enactment, and the achievement of conflict. *Contemporary Psychoanalysis, 40,* 197–237.

Wachtel, P. (2008). *Relational theory and the practice of psychotherapy.* New York: Guilford.

Chapter 6

Myths about empathy and mirror neurons

Empathy continues to be an overburdened concept, having been defined and redefined countless times. Yet its prominence is retained because it endures as an essential factor in positive therapeutic outcome. The latest research on mirror neurons has been partially misapplied to the notion of empathy, positing that there is evidence that we are hardwired to be objectively empathic, meaning that there will be little to no difference between what the patient is feeling and what we feel. Although the literature *does* confirm the greater likelihood of persons in positive relationships being more open and likely to feeling each other's emotions, there is no evidence that this is primarily a result of mirror neuron activity. Furthermore, there are many variables that affect not only the extent that empathy is felt but also the types of feelings and actions that follow.

The assumption that the analyst's experience of empathy routinely produces a therapeutic response is essentially false. This chapter explores the neuroscience research that has been misapplied in the therapy relationship, while using this and other research to explain the function of empathy in the therapeutic process. Further, I want to tie our preoccupation with empathy into the theme of this volume by examining how and why we find the idea of being effortlessly empathic so appealing. This includes a discussion of why we cannot be consistently empathic; how differing definitions of what constitutes empathy detract from meaningful dialogue; why empathy does not necessarily lead to compassionate action; and how we have misunderstood and misapplied the concept of mirror neurons in our pursuit of unattainable synchrony with the other.

The mirror neuron controversy

The analytic world has become "infatuated" (Vivona, 2009a) with the concept of mirror neurons. The analytic focus on mirror neurons relies on the disputed belief that humans naturally and automatically feel what someone else is feeling, and that this phenomenon is hardwired in our brains. Though not a neuroscientist myself, I have long worked to stay informed about basic neuroscience research and have applied it frequently in my previous writing. Unlike some of my analytic colleagues (Blass & Carmeli, 2007, Pulver, 2003), I believe that neuroscience has much to offer us, both in theoretical and clinical applications.

Nonetheless, it is hard to disagree with those who say that our application of the mirror neuron discovery is at best premature, and at worst an undermining of basic analytic concepts, interventions, and principles of scientific inference. Hickock (2014), in his provocatively titled book *The Myth of Mirror Neurons*, provides an excellent overview of the neuroscience findings on mirror neurons in language any analyst can understand. He echoes Vivona's (2009a) dismay at the worldwide hype about mirror neurons as he attempts to set the record straight.

Yes, mirror neurons do exist. But the meaning of their name and function has been greatly exaggerated. Even mirror neuron theorists like Gallese et al. (2007) state that the very concept of mirroring is "misleading." And Vivona (2009a) says, "Despite their name, most mirror neurons do not match or mirror, but instead fire in response to a range of similar observed actions (Rizzolatti & Craighero, 2004, Csibra, 2004)" (p. 536). Thus, the fact that we do respond at numerous levels, both in and out of awareness, is not in dispute. But the importance of mirror neurons in determining what we feel and how we respond certainly is.

How mirror neuron theory began

Hickock (2014) explains that a group of neuroscientists in Parma, Italy, headed by Giacomo Rizzolatti, were working on an experiment with macaque monkeys, having implanted microelectrode probes in their brains. They observed firing in certain cells as the monkeys grasped an object. They also noted that the cells that fired differed based on the size of the object and occurred even when the object was simply there to be seen. The researchers' main discovery, dubbed "mirror neurons," occurred accidentally as the experimenters swapped out objects and moved around the room. The monkeys were still being monitored and—lo and behold—they saw the monkeys' neurons fire in a way that matched the movements of the experimenters. Thus, they discovered that macaque monkeys' neurons fired in a pattern that was the same both when they reached and grasped and when they observed another monkey or human reaching or grasping. Mirror neuron theory was thus born.

Rizzolatti and his colleague Michael Arbit (1998) published one paper about their discoveries entitled "Language within Our Grasp," which Hickock (2014) says "proposed that mirror neurons may unlock the secrets of language" (p. 21). In the same year (1998) another of their collaborators, Vittoria Gallese, and his philosopher colleague Alvin Godman, published a paper called "Mirror Neurons and the Simulation Theory of Mind-Reading." It is not hard to see why Hickok, or any person trained in research methods and reporting, would question the validity of making these huge inferences about the human mind from the results of a study revealing monkeys' ability to view and imitate the simple grasping of objects. The data simply are not there.

Hickok makes it clear that he does not really dispute the results of the Parma group's original study, describing the patterns of neurons that fire in response to monkeys' actions and anticipation or viewing of certain actions. (He admits to being deliberately hyperbolic in titling his book.) Nor does he doubt that we have similar reactions in our human brains. As a cognitive scientist, what bothers him is the overextension of these results. It appears that with the mirror neuron experiments in hand, both the initial researchers themselves, as well as psychoanalysts, social psychologists, and the media, have suggested that mirror neurons are the basis for action understanding (e.g., why did the person reach out at this moment), as well as the basis for empathy and intention-reading—all based on unconfirmed hypotheses about mirror neurons in humans.

It is hard to argue with the position that the reach of mirror neuron research has—if you excuse the pun—exceeded its grasp. Hickok (2014) says, "By the mid-2000s, the theory had morphed from 'speculation' (to use the mirror neuron discoverers' own words) to a 'virtual theoretical fortress'" (p. 7). Hickok believes that the extreme popularity of mirror neuron theories has to do with their simplicity, bringing rather simple, straightforward explanations to complex topics, and offering neurobiology as proof. Illustrating the faulty logic in extending mirror neuron firings in monkeys to human language, he humorously asks, "If mirror resonance is the basis of human language, why don't macaques talk?" (p. 227). (One could add, "Why can't they recognize themselves in a mirror, like chimpanzees?)

Without burdening the analytic reader with an undue amount of neuroscience reporting, suffice it to say that one of the main issues facing the identification of mirror neurons and their functions in the human brain is that we cannot implant electrodes in human subjects, as was done with the macaque monkeys. We mostly rely on various fMRI imaging techniques and their interpretations instead. And variations in study design make comparisons difficult.

Are the researchers truly researching the same phenomenon in their attempt to validate the existence of mirror neurons in humans or not? Even when research protocols are similar, results to date have been inconclusive at best, invalidating at worst, depending on your perspective. More importantly, even if we *could* easily replicate the original studies on mirror neurons in humans, we would still fall far short of using these results as confirmation of undistorted empathy and its correlates.

Does mirror neuron theory predict empathy?

The application of mirror neuron theory in psychology, psychoanalysis, and social-cognitive neuroscience has focused on both identifying a neural basis for empathy and then concluding how it operates within human relationships. However, this endeavor has proved to be elusive at best. A recent research report by Bolding (2019) sums up the repeated failure to establish mirror neurons in humans, particularly as they relate to the experience of empathy. She appears to think that much of the mirror neuron research devoted to empathy is premature, putting the proverbial cart before the horse.

[E]ven if a functional link exists, the MNS (Mirror Neuron System) cannot be the only neural mechanism underlying empathy. Nevertheless, fundamental evidence of a MNS in the human brain must first be found, before chasing hard evidence for the MSN-empathy link. (p. 9)

In a recent meta-analysis of the literature by Bekkali et al. (2020), they were a bit more convinced of mirror neuron patterns in humans yet were even more skeptical about their primacy in empathy. They say that some research suggests that "MNS could be extended to emotional domain (Christov-Moore et al., 2014)," but quickly added that "this does not mean the MNS is the only implementer of empathy" (p. 5). In other words, the claims about primacy appear to be overstated and/or premature. But the claims about MNS involvement in empathy might have some scientific merit.

They state further that the literature ultimately provides more evidence for empathy as a socially learned[1] and variable response rather than one that is primarily hardwired. In fact, they point out several studies showing that there can be empathy without any visual cues, such as when listening to a sad song or reading stories about another's painful feelings. They conclude that the mirror neuron system in empathy "can be set as the reproduction of affective experience of others in your own repertoire, but there is still not enough empirical evidence to conclude a causal link between the MNS and empathy" (p. 9).

Neuroscientists will tell you that most brain functions involve activity across different areas of the brain, which can limit the validity and generalizability of any study focused on a single area (McGilchrist, 2010). Zaki and Ochsner (2012) note how limited the enormous body of research on empathy is, due to this narrow focus on a studying a single word or facial expression. Multiple definitions of empathy and the single facet approach to most research studies generate varied results that fall short of a meaningful assessment of what happens between two people. The authors liken this to drawing inferences about the sound of an orchestra while listening to only one of the instruments.

These research results are not exhaustive, of course. But my point is to sufficiently challenge the notion of applying mirror neuron research to broader and more complex human interactions. I think we also have to question our motivations regarding our own desires to rescue and be rescued, how the notion of an idealized, presymbolic merger is part of that fantasy, and how we are quick to embrace theories that create the possibility of this occurring.

The psychanalytic position on mirror neurons

One can see the appeal of automatic "brain to brain" communication of emotion, unscathed by bias and perception. It implies an almost effortless, and extremely effective, communication between any two people who are engaged with each other. Only emotional contagion, which is unconscious, approaches this standard. But even emotional contagion is not a given; we can, and do, put up barriers to receiving other's emotions. Plus, we do not yet understand the brain functions that are responsible for emotional contagion. As Barrett (2017) points out,

> Even after a century of effort, scientific research has not revealed a consistent, physical fingerprint for even a single emotion. When scientists attach electrodes to a person's face and measure how facial muscles actually move during the experience of an emotion, they find tremendous variety, not uniformity. (p. xii)

In psychoanalysis, the application of mirror neuron research has gone far beyond emotional contagion. Rather, it is sometimes elevated to a theory of mind, attempting to substantiate the existence of complex, unbiased, automatic, complementary emotional responses. But is this even remotely possible? The Boston Change Process Study Group has been a particularly strong and convincing advocate for the idea of this type of sophisticated unconscious-to-unconscious communication of affect and intentions, based partially on this concept of automatic affective mirroring. A longtime critique of this application, Vivona (2009a) says,

> In this model, the analyst's brain provides a version of patient experience, minimally influenced by the analyst's psychology, which might be accessed for understanding the patient. *The biological purity of this mechanism is appealing as it posits a direct and accurate path to knowing the patient, a new royal road to the unconscious mind of the*

other. This interpretation of mirror neuron research is consistent with a growing position with contemporary psychoanalysis that important interpersonal processes operate outside awareness and that verbal involvement in these processes is both infrequent and unnecessary (e.g., Boston Change Process Study Group, 2005; for a critique, see Vivona, 2006). (p. 541, emphasis added)

Vivona has challenged the idea that we could essentially remove verbalization and insight from the analytic process, relying instead on unconscious communication. In addition to her criticism of the Boston Change Process Study Group, she debated with mirror neuron theorists in the pages of the *Journal of the American Psychoanalytic Association* in 2009, citing numerous problems with the applications of mirror neuron theory, as well as unquestioning acceptance of both its role in emotional communication and its relevance for psychoanalysis.

She challenges what she sees as unvalidated assumptions made by Gallese et al. (2007). The first she calls the "Correspondence Assumption," meaning that we are assuming that if we know something about what is going on in the brain, we know what is happening in the mind. There is simply no evidence for this. The second is the "Shared Experience Assumption": "This is the assumption that similar brain activity in the observer and in the one who is observed indicates a similar internal experience of the two individuals" (p. 532). This builds on the first assumption, again without any evidence. Her third assumption, the "Directness Assumption," centers on believing that it is possible for there to be a pure communication between two individuals based on extending from brain to mind: "At the very least, conscious and unconscious expectations, linguistic categories, and personal memories infuse our observations of others (Barrett, 2017) and therefore conspire to shape any simulation of those observations" (p. 544). In addition to quoting the burgeoning literature that contests the role of mirror neurons and their importance in empathy, she notes that our responses to others' pain is often not congruent with what that person is feeling, a topic I will take up in the next section of this chapter on the limits of empathy.

Eagle et al. (2009, which includes Gallese) responded to Vivona's criticisms in the same journal issue and were surprisingly receptive to her thesis. At the outset, they say, "We agree that the premature or simplistic importation of neuroscience findings into psychoanalysis is ill-advised and only pseudoscientific" (p. 559). They also agree that any thought of a pure transfer of feelings from one person to another is not justified and that "embodied simulation and cognitive inferential processes are necessary for understanding the other" (p. 566). (However, the Boston Change Process Study Group, 2018, does advocate for this type of direct link, a topic I will explore further in the next chapter on therapeutic action.)

Eagle et al. also had points of disagreement, of course. Their primary criticism of Vivona has to do with her insistence that mirror neurons have not been proven to exist in humans. Vivona has altered that view, in light of the fact that mirror neurons were subsequently located in humans. She notes, however, that their location in the brain did not match the theory (Vivona, personal communication).

In spite of the increasing evidence for the existence of mirror neurons in humans, the argument still stands that there has been no evidence for mirror neurons having a primary role in empathy, emotional contagion, or even facial mimicry. As Hickock (2014) points out, "Paradoxically, unconscious mimicry is, in fact, highly selective. Humans tend to imitate people they like and distinctly avoid imitating people they don't like" (p. 203).

Mirror neurons are some of the many neurons that fire during our interactive responses and do not account for the wide individual differences that have been reported. The majority of researchers agree that there is much more research that needs to be done Bekkali et al. (2020), along with better techniques for neuroimaging in humans, before we can have any real idea of what is happening in the brain during emotional communication.

I agree with Vivona that the Boston Change Process Study Group, who has been enormously influential, is essentially making questionable inferences from Rizzolatti & Sinigaglia, 2008) original research to complex human responses. Citing Rizzolatti et al., they draw the following unsupported conclusion.

Thus, the same area of the brain that facilitates our physical act of grasping underlies our intuitive grasp of others' intentions. It is no accident that we speak of "getting" another person, or of someone important who "gets me," in the sense of relating to me in a deeply satisfying way. (p. 744)

The "grasp" that the BCPSG is talking about, as emphasized here, is literally a basic motor activity observed in monkeys. Even though it has been tentatively confirmed in human beings, it has not been proven to be the basis of our "grasping" others' intentions, which is a complex activity of the mind. This remains true even if mirror neurons are involved in some way. Lamm and Majdandzic (2015) say, "In general, it seems unlikely that mirror neuron responses serve as input to contribute to high-level intention understanding (Csibra, 2008, Hickok, 2009, Uithol et al., 2011)" (p. 20). The key term here is "high-level intention."

When we talk about intentions in human behavior, we are not referring to the ability to anticipate the grasping and lifting of an object; we are talking about human motivations for behaviors and attitudes. To equate these is misleading. Arizmendi (2011) discusses this controversy surrounding the generalization of motor activities to higher systems in the brain, involving such concepts as desires and beliefs. And as McGilchrist (2010) points out,

Imaging just shows a few peaks, where much of interest goes on elsewhere. One cannot assume that the areas that light up are those fundamentally responsible for the "function" being imaged, or that areas that do not light up are not involved. (p. 35)

Vivona (2009b) makes the point that she is not against neuroscience—quite the opposite—and I find myself in the same camp. I am fascinated by neuroscience and look forward to continued research and thoughts regarding implications for analytic treatment. But when it comes to unconscious to unconscious communication, that day awaits us. "As we consider the wealth of ideas in a field like neuroscience, it is important to recognize that connections between the scientific data are *constructed* by psychoanalysts, not *demonstrated* by researchers" (p. 1354).

Although the misapplication of neuroscience has been attributed to our desire to be seen as "scientists" (Brothers, 2002) and to be fascinated by new theories in general (think about the many analytic presentations that took place on "chaos theory" and "string theory," for example), I think our motivations go beyond this. Our desire to embrace a seemingly magical and effortless route to another's emotions may well have more do with our need to be the perfect mother/analyst. We want to believe that a direct, uninfluenced path to another's feelings is possible.

I think the "why" of this is complex, but it is not difficult to understand why we would embrace an almost magical path between ourselves and our patients. It reduces the possibility of our making serious therapeutic errors as long as we are open to our patients' emotions. Perhaps it also gives us needed hope and the excitement that comes with new ideas. What we all experience every day is both the rewards of affective attunement when we feel it, but also the frustrations that routinely arise as we, along with our patients, fail to achieve this.

Restating some of the themes of this book, I think we may also be enthralled with an unconscious-to-unconscious process as the guiding force in treatment because it relieves us of some of the burdensome responsibility we feel for "fixing" people; it allows us to avoid confrontation as we await enactment. We can justify being passive and feel a certain "innocence" regarding ensuing conflict if it arises through mutual projective identification rather that direct confrontation, as stated in the previous chapter.

The simple truth is that really understanding what another person is feeling, being able to hold and regulate that feeling—especially if it is painful or alienating—and then respond constructively is quite difficult. One of my supervisees recently told me that she thought she was quite good at empathizing and accepting feelings (which she is) and also good at thinking about her patients intellectually (also true), but she responded with a bit of dismay when I told her the challenge was to do them both at once. "How is that even possible?" she said. I said it was more a matter of rapidly switching back and forth between those two modalities to create an integrated perspective from which to intervene. So it is not hard to understand why therapists would welcome the possibility of easing our burden through relying on an unconscious process to guide us.

The problems with empathy

We have at least two significant problems regarding empathy in psychoanalysis. One, we are too concerned with feeling what the patient feels and endorsing those feelings. Two, we do not have a shared definition of empathy, either as a single emotion-based in-the-moment response or in the greater context of what constitutes empathic interventions. Certainly, we all work to establish a good working relationship with our patients by expressing our genuine curiosity and sensitivity to what they have suffered or are suffering. But over time, as I (and Hirsch, 2008) have suggested previously, do we maintain this attempt at empathic "holding" for too long? And what is too long? One common instance of "too long," is long after either patient or analyst have ceased to feel emotion when the patient recites his woes.

This section of the chapter is devoted to discussing how empathy works or does not work in analytic treatment and in all relationships. I want to utilize some of the research on empathy from other disciplines to help sort out a working definition of empathy, and I want to further discuss the limits of our empathy and the implications for doing treatment.

One of the key problems in both researching what we call empathy and discussing it clinically is the tremendous variation in how it is defined. I think we need to make the distinction in psychoanalysis that is made in the broader social psychology and neuroscience literature on the definition of empathy, especially regarding its basic functions. Empathy and sympathy (with prosocial behavior) are different; one does not necessarily follow from the other. To help clarify some of the misconceptions surrounding the concept of empathy, I want to not only review the relevant literature but also provide a working definition. Arizmendi (2011) provides the following:

> Despite the fact that researchers do not always agree on the definition of empathy, virtually all researchers, theorists, and clinicians agree that it extends beyond emotional synchrony or attunement to another person (Stern, 1985, Rizzolatti & Sinigaglia 2008, Damasio, 2003). In fact, empathy is typically thought to include both an emotional resonance and a cognitive component. (p. 409)

Noted neuroscience researcher Decety (2010), along with many others, distinguishes between empathy and sympathy. (This distinction is not made in psychoanalysis, where the term *empathy* most often assumes a responding posture in the analyst of both shared affect and subsequent deep listening and prosocial behavior.) Decety says empathy and sympathy are often confused and offers this simple distinction: "I distinguish between empathy, simply defined as the ability to recognize the emotions and feelings of others with a minimal distinction between self and other, and sympathy, i.e., feelings of concern about the welfare of others" (p. 258).

Hein and Singer (2008) make further distinctions, noting the differences between empathy, sympathy, and emotional contagion.

> [E]mpathy is not necessarily linked to a prosocial motivation, that is, the concern about the others' wellbeing, whereas there is such a link from sympathy or compassion to prosociality...Lastly empathy has to be separated from emotional contagion. Empathy involves awareness. Emotional contagion might be a precursor for empathy, but is not considered an empathic response, because the person incorporates affective states of another person without being aware that it is not his own feeling. (p. 154)

I think this clarification is potentially helpful both for better definition in analytic theory and in the discussion of countertransference. We need to make room for understanding that what Hein and Singer and others are talking about when they say that feeling another's emotions does not necessarily lead to a helpful response from the other, and, perhaps more crucial to this discussion, the cognitive processes involved in truly understanding another's intentions and needs involves different neural networks.

To summarize, the tasks involved in what is commonly referred to as "empathy" in psychoanalysis are comprised of three different but related activities: first, the communication of affect from one person to another; second, the subsequent emotional and cognitive responding to that affect; and third, by subsequent behavioral responses. The assumption in treatment is that these responses will be sympathetic and helpful (prosocial).

As stated, instead of assuming that we are mostly empathic in the sense that we respond directly to another's feelings with a mirrored version of those feelings, we could benefit from a more nuanced and accurate definition that recognizes the unconscious emotional communication along with both our complex emotional and cognitive responses. Again, our tendency to focus on early childhood as a model for analytic treatment fails us. Babies and very young children rely heavily on facial mimicry. But as our brains develop, the cognitive aspects of our responding become more complex and idiosyncratic. Decety and Michalski (2010), in researching developmental changes in the brain, report that

> This pattern of functional changes supports the general notion that the development of affective processing from childhood to adulthood is accompanied by reduced activity within limbic affect processing systems, and increased involvement of other prefrontal systems (Killgore & Yurgelun-Todd, 2007). Watching someone in pain elicits a negative arousal response in the observers, to a stronger degree in children than in young adults. (pp. 895–896)

Thus, the extension of early mother/infant communication becomes increasingly oversimplistic when talking about adult to adult communication of any kind, and it notably skews in the direction of underestimating the adult patient.

The patient who on one day inspires tender feelings and a strong desire to understand and help may on another day evoke little or no feeling in the analyst. Or he or she may stimulate anxiety, hopelessness—even disgust. These differences cannot be ascribed to the patient alone, of course. They have very much to do with the current feeling states of the analyst, as well as his or her values, cultural background, past experiences, and sensitivities to certain issues. And, as the above quoted literature indicates, even if we experience the patient's feelings much the same as he does, there is no guarantee we will be receptive and sympathetic to those feelings. The kind of empathy analysts aspire to is exactly that—an aspiration.

Nonetheless, if viewed within the realm of our human limitations, empathy—the tolerance and acceptance of that empathically received

emotion, the ability to tolerate and process our own subsequent reactions, and the ability to respond constructively—is what treatment
is about. Rather than assume that we all are mostly empathic, I prefer
to look at what the research says along with what we know from our
own clinical experience, then accept and teach those realities to
trainees.

I think the stereotype of the endlessly empathic analyst belies the
reality that a true empathic response often involves either a reframing
of the patient's experience or a confrontation of some sort, a point
made by Kohut (1971). Passively feeling what the patient is feeling (to
the extent this is possible) may lead to the patient initially feeling
cared about and accepted, but it may still fall short of what the patient needs. This is especially true over time. Experienced analysts
know this, of course, but I do not think it is frequently taught in these
terms, mostly because it begs for examples of what analysts do, which
we are reluctant to disclose. What follows is a case example that illustrates these concepts in a basic, brief format.

The case of Sarah

Sarah, a 40-something mother of two, began treatment due to anxiety
and depression surrounding her marriage and the sexual abuse of her
youngest daughter. These topics were intertwined because the sexual
abuse was committed by a nephew on her husband's side of the family.
Another family member walked in unexpectedly during sexual activity,
put a stop to it, and informed Sarah and her husband. Sarah expressed
severe guilt over not guessing that the abuse was taking place, given that
her daughter had had an unexplained vaginal infection.

Sarah also wondered aloud if she was not just like her mother, who
looked the other way when Sarah's brother was sadistically teasing
her, dominating her, approaching her in her bed, and touching her in
the middle of the night. After many years of this, Sarah finally told
her father, who was shocked and took Sarah's brother aside immediately to put a stop to it.

Sarah said, given her own history, she should have known something was going on. In reality, her daughter was only four at the time
the abuse began, and she was gradually indoctrinated rather than
being sexually assaulted. This went on for three years.

Sarah feels this blame has inevitably leaked into her marriage, even though her husband quickly condemned his nephew's actions. She and her husband have no social contact with this part of the family, but her husband still occasionally speaks to his brother, who is the abuser's father. As the parent of the abuser, he says he still cannot believe that it really took place and that if it did, that his son was the perpetrator.

Sarah repeatedly said she also felt guilty that she could not forgive her nephew for his actions. Given his young age, she wonders if he was simply repeating something that was done to him, the implication being that she is unjustly blaming the victim. She said she feels like a bad person because it has been six years since the transgression was discovered and she is still so upset. And her marriage is deteriorating. Doesn't this make her a bad person?

I listened to this story being replayed many times and was always empathic and encouraging of Sarah to accept her anger and not be so hard on herself. I have told her that it is exceedingly difficult to forgive someone who has not admitted to wrongdoing and is not seeking forgiveness. This always seems to comfort her in the moment, yet she inevitably returned to this scenario with accompanying deep pain and anger. As I have said in my writing many times, when a patient keeps repeating an emotional scenario, without any dilution in its intensity, I know the patient is coming back because she still needs some kind of response that I have failed to deliver.

One day as Sarah repeated this scenario, I realized that with every iteration of this story, I feel her intense pain and anger. She uses the couch and presumably does not see that I sometimes tear up when she tells this story. What I also feel is intense outrage at what happened to her young daughter. And I could not help but notice that I never failed to feel this, and feel it deeply, each time Sarah revisited it. In addition to feeling her hurt and anger, I also imagined wanting to hurt her nephew. I was curious about my reaction, given that I am not prone to hostility. But then guilt and shame about these thoughts would creep in, and I would shake them off. Eventually, I began to stay with this fantasy and wonder if there was any possible way to express what I was thinking and feeling in a way that would be helpful to Sarah. I also wondered how appropriate it was to go in this direction when her stated goal was to mitigate rather than intensify her anger.

Finally, I decided to simply tell her what came to mind. As she talked about the rape of her daughter, I felt rage bubbling up in me and said, "I know you would like to forgive your nephew, but if someone did what he did to a child of mine, I would want to kill him." With that, she began to sob, which she had not done before. She spent the next ten minutes that were left in her session crying and saying how hard it was. Then, as she got up to leave, she turned to me and said, "Thank you."

It became apparent in future sessions that my willingness to acknowledge the possibility of murderous rage, not just in her, but in myself, was immensely relieving for Sarah. Her guilt and shame were ameliorated almost immediately, and this issue began to recede as a focal point of her treatment narrative. This was not an issue in my life, but the repetitive empathic immersion in Sarah's experience allowed me to feel and to name her emotional experience. More importantly, convinced of her underlying rage and the guilt and shame associated with those feelings, I was able to not only empathize but also to speak for her in a way that was freeing and validating. I verbalized not her guilt and shame over lack of forgiveness, but rather her murderous rage.

An important point I want to make here is that when Sarah first began treatment, I never would have dreamed of making this kind of intervention. There must be an existing attachment in a safe setting to say this kind of thing. And the education I received over time, as she occasionally repeated the story, helped me to better understand what both of us were feeling. Gradually, I began to think more about what I could say while I was in the midst of feeling strongly, and how I would say it. I knew I had to say what I was thinking with emotion in my voice or it would not be effective.

I think my intervention illustrates that basic empathy—just sharing her feeling and letting her know I was (both by my empathic statements and facial expression) was all she initially needed, and therefore was therapeutic. But that is one of the fascinating challenges of doing analytic work—following the patient's lead and becoming aware when the situation is morphing into something else, something that needs a new, more creative and personal response.

Sometimes, it calls for a deeper interpretation; often, it requires an emotional disclosure—one that is carefully crafted, yet authentic in the moment. Simply staying with, and feeling, her guilt, shame, and grief were helpful to her, but she let me know by her repetition of the scenario that she needed something more. I think this case illustrates the potential evolutionary aspect of empathy within the analytic relationship as treatment progresses. It also illustrates the aforementioned three-prong composition of what has been defined here as empathy: shared affect, cognitive processing and assessment, and positive intervention.

However, empathy alone has its limitations, including not always being possible. In the next section of this chapter, I want to return to the research on empathy to discuss these limitations and their potential impact on treatment.

The limitations of empathy

To begin, we need to disabuse ourselves of the notion that empathy, as well as its cognitive and behavioral correlates (e.g., sympathetic concern and prosocial behavior), is easily accomplished, let alone automatic. As human beings, we are more empathic toward people who are similar to us and people we like. And if something is painful for another but would not be painful for us, our responses will be weak or nonexistent.

Even when the conditions for empathy have been met, studies on empathy have demonstrated that truly being empathic, in the three-step process outlined above, is quite selective. Human beings routinely respond to other's expression of distress with their own *personal distress*. Personal distress arises with shared pain and often results in a nonhelpful response. Although this concept is well researched and written about in related disciplines, it is almost nonexistent in the analytic literature.

Notable exceptions are Vivona's (2009b) excellent piece, cited earlier, and one by Knox (2013). Knox provides an in-depth discussion of the need for some type of identification, often referred to as "trial identification" in the analytic literature, as part of the empathic process. But she also warns that overidentification is a primary source of analyst masochism or withdrawal, particularly with trauma patients. She cites the neuroscience literature to make the point of the need for the clinician's ability to distance enough to gain a perspective.

> [W]itnessing someone else's emotions could, for example, result, purely, in personal distress and a self-centered response in the observer. So empathy also depends on cognitive processes of perspective taking and executive control: which allows individuals to be aware of their intentions and feelings and to maintain separate perspectives on self and other...knowing whose action (including emotions) belongs to whom preserves individuals from over-identifying with the observed target, which would otherwise lead to empathic distress (Decety & Meyer, 2009, p. 144) (p. 493).

The notion of feeling the patient's personal distress is certainly not new, nor is the possibility of countertransference responses to that distress that might result in ill-advised actions. What is missing in the analytic literature, and therefore mostly absent in analytic training, is the concept of personal distress as ongoing, especially with patients who have been traumatized; the need for a certain degree of vigilance for maintaining needed psychic separation; and the inescapable truth that we are not above the human need to relieve our own distress. A recent study by Kim and Han (2018) confirmed Batson's (1987) early work on how the listener's degree of personal distress interferes with empathy.

Therefore, another type of vigilance is required when asking whether an intervention is aimed primarily at relieving the patient's distress or one's own. As someone who has advocated for judicious self-disclosure for almost 30 years, I frankly admit some analysts use this intervention for relieving their own distress more than the patient's. I have had other analysts tell me how much they admire my work, then go on to relay a story of their self-disclosure that made me cringe. I realize that these errors are inevitable and that I certainly have made my share, but if we have any hopes of creating new types of interventions, we need both a theory that explains them and serious discussion about parameters.

Accepting the normal ambivalent reaction to the patient's personal distress would also help to reduce guilt and shame over our sometime desire to squash that distress or flee. One of the most frequent complaints I have heard from patients who had some previous treatment that they were dissatisfied with revolved around their therapists talking too much or being too silent. Sitting with another person's intense emotional pain is far more difficult than the way we portray it in our case presentations. Goubert et al. (2009) report some common reactions.

> In some instances, therefore, observers who respond with high distress to the perception of another individual in pain might be motivated to underestimate the observed person's pain, in an attempt to keep their own distress within acceptable limits (Goubert et al., 2005) or to constrain the other's pain-related emotional expression (Herbette & Rimé, 2004) (p. 156).

I think as analysts we are more inclined to constrain our patients' pain-related expressions as we rush to be a soothing presence, including quickly apologizing for any role we might have in their pain. Doing so, of course, succeeds in truncating the patient's pain, but also forecloses the deeper exploration and meaning of that pain.

We routinely idealize our empathic capacities, which can create a problem in and of itself. From my experience in both listening to case presentations and reading accounts in the literature, current notions of right-brain-to-right-brain communication of affect tilt noticeably toward symbiotic merger under the aegis of affective communication. These theories are akin to Gallese et al.'s (2007) embodied simulation theory of mirror neurons. The literature on empathy, however, warns against this stance as ideal for producing needed cognitive assessments and subsequent prosocial behavior. Noted empathy researcher Batson (2009) states plainly,

> Feeling as the other feels may actually inhibit other-oriented feelings if it leads us to become focused on our own emotional state. Sensing the nervousness of other passengers on an airplane in rough weather, I too may become nervous. If I focus on my own nervousness, not theirs, I am likely to feel less for them, not more. (p. 10)

I have supervised therapists who are in the habit of sharing not only feelings but also life experiences with their patients. Sometimes, they verbalize it to the patient; at other times, they simply verbalized it to themselves or me. Nonetheless, I have always discouraged this type of response, instead urging them to focus on the patient as much as possible, forgoing the need for identification, and inquiring as to their preference for it. So I was quite interested when I read the following from social neuroscience researchers Decety and Lamm (2009):

> The frontal lobes may functionally serve to separate perspectives, helping one to resist interference from one's own perspective when adopting the subjective perspective of another (Decety & Jackson, 2004). This ability is of particular importance when observing another's distress, because a complete merging with the target would lead to confusion as to who is experiencing the negative emotions and therefore to different motivations as to who should be the target of supportive behavior. (p. 204)

Hence, our desires to both merge with our patients and also decouple from them. Some degree of merger is necessary for shared affective experience yet too much can erase the boundaries between patient and analyst.

So what makes for successful empathic experience, meaning shared affect, cognitive appraisal, and subsequent prosocial (helping) behavior? Unsurprisingly, it is the listener's ability to self-regulate, including the ability to maintain the aforementioned level of separateness. Self-regulation is stronger in adults than it is in children (Rothbart et al., 1994, Zelazo et al., 2004), having been documented as a developmental task. And "compassion training" like the Buddhist meditation "Loving Kindness" (Lamm & Majdandzic, 2015) has been shown effective in increasing self-regulation and accompanying acceptance and prosocial interventions. Additional research has demonstrated that "compassion training" has also been effective in increasing the capacity for empathy (Engen & Singer, 2015).

Certainly, this bodes well for therapists having higher levels of empathy, since we have, in a sense, received our early training as family caregivers, and our years of analytic training have enhanced those natural compassion skills.

The challenge to be empathic

Nevertheless, we necessarily struggle at times to be empathic, particularly when we are being criticized or blamed for the patient's pain. As hard as we might try to avoid this, our responses to our patients' negative emotions are often some form of distancing or rejection. We infrequently discuss the reality of not wanting to share our patients' negative feelings, let alone feeling disgust, anger, or other negative emotions in response. But we do feel these things. Vivona (2009a) reports research findings from a study done by Schulte-Ruther et al. (2007), where subjects were shown static images depicting facial expressions of anger and fear. Although they accurately identified these expressions, the subjects' own emotional experience was often different, thereby defying the "shared experience" assumption. She reports that

> Emotional responses to the fearful facial expressions revealed a mixture of congruent (e.g., "afraid") and reactive (e.g., "compassionate") emotions, whereas, responses to the angry facial expressions were overwhelmingly reactive; most participant reported such reactive feelings as "attacked," "uneasy," or "uncomfortable," and very few reported such congruent feelings as "aggressive" or "irritated." (pp. 537–538)

I think this explains why we have so much difficulty with our negative countertransference. In spite of the research saying it is perfectly normal to react negatively to another person's aggressive feelings and statements, we somehow think we should be "above" these normal responses. Our guilt and shame about reacting negatively to our patients creates fertile ground for inauthentic responses and discourages the development of constructive approaches to dealing with negative emotions.

We are in the habit of denying our capacity for aggression, let alone pettiness or a desire to act out hostility toward our patients. The literature states that when people are in competition, empathy goes out the window (Lanzetta & Englis, 1989). Granted, this study was done with people in aggressive competitive relationships, not in therapy. Yet it makes sense that during power struggles or emotional threats, empathy would be in short supply. Patients with narcissistic personalities are known for their need to stimulate envy in others, including their therapists. They make not so subtle references to being superior (e.g., wealthier, more successful, or more intelligent than the analyst). Yet it would be unheard of to admit to experiencing schadenfreude when such a patient suffers some minor comeuppance. These are the things we dare not discuss. Equally verboten are our feelings of disgust and repugnance.

I recall treating a very disturbed young woman fairly early in my career who I will call Sheila. Sheila found it terribly difficult to connect with anyone. Only in her 20s, she had been in therapy three times per week with analysts since the age of 14. It became clear that she relied on therapy as a form of companionship and had a questionable prognosis from the outset. Nonetheless, I took her on at the urging of the referring analyst from another state.

Sheila was deeply introverted and spent all of her time outside of work alone. Tiring of empathic remarks and interpretations, she would plead with me for advice on how to be more social. She claimed she lacked these skills and needed to discuss possible activities to do on the weekend. When I would reluctantly agree to do this, we would come up with a plan that she seemed enthusiastic about. However, every Monday she would come to her session and report that she had not left the house other than to let her dog out. As she reported her "failure" to me, a slight smirk often registered on her face. When I asked her about her facial expression, she simply denied it.

It became clear, however, that she had not made much progress in her lifelong treatment because of her need to defeat anyone who attempted to break into her emotional isolation and influence her. As I mentioned earlier in this book, we both wished to influence each other, as naturally occurs. What became clear over time was that she was winning. I was becoming listless and depressed in her sessions. And I was also beginning to resent her. The more I resented her, the worse I felt about myself as a therapist.

Finally, after months with no progress whatsoever, she came to her Monday session and said she had done something she was ashamed of. She wanted to tell me but was afraid I would be disgusted. I told her that we would work through anything she had to say. Then she looked at me with that same smirk and told me that she had put food on her labia and had her dog lick it off.

In that moment I felt total disgust. I kept telling myself that I should not—that therapists weren't supposed to feel that way and that she was counting on me not to feel disgusted. She then asked me if I did. I thought for a moment and told her I was a bit shocked. I hadn't expected what she revealed to me. Then I assured her I could work through that and I emphasized her feelings of loneliness and desperation as motivation for her behavior. (This is an example of the "pseudo-empathy" I discuss later.) I do not recall there being much that occurred following that event.

That treatment occurred too long ago to know how I might have handled the situation better, given the treatment approach I have used for more than 30 years. But in retrospect, she may have wanted me to be disgusted and perhaps more honest about it. But I often find this excuse to be rather flimsy when I hear other clinicians offer it up, so I am equally skeptical of my motivations for doing so. I do not know for sure what was happening in the bigger picture of our ongoing relationship, but I know I felt disgusted and confused. And I wished that there had been some context for me to comprehend that experience, other than feeling inadequate and lacking in proper empathy.

Beyond empathy

Just as with many of the topics in this volume, the study of empathy had its heyday in the 1970s and 1980s. Our ability to go "beyond empathy," by which I mean taking the next step after incorporating the two-person perspective with empathic understanding and internal responding, has lagged considerably. Instead, we have embraced theories that create a greater sense of "not knowing" (Boston Change Process Study Group, 2005) and rely on unconscious processes rather than deliberate action. I find it odd that despite the original goal of analysis being "making the unconscious, conscious," we now focus on an analytic experience that may or may not include insight.

Possibly appealing to the analyst's fears of doing harm and companion fear of conflict, as well as playing to the strengths we exhibited in our families of origin (empathy and soothing), analytic treatment has arguably never been a more passive activity. Bolognini

(1997, 2001) has been an outspoken critic of our strong emphasis on empathy as a primary intervention. He says,

> On the clinical level, the idea that the analyst must deliberately seek to empathize with the patient is stated to have gained currency, but the author argues that such an attempt to achieve empathy by force can lead only to "empathism," which is a dogmatic, hyperconcordant attitude whereby the inexperienced analyst in particular thinks he can control the process better. (1997, p. 279)

He also cites Manfredi Turillazzi (1994), who discusses how the analyst can use "empathy" as a way of over-identifying with the patient, gratifying his own needs and desires and avoiding pain. If the reader recalls, this resembles Mitchell's early objections to the emphasis on the "developmental tilt" discussed in the previous chapter.

In spite of these warnings, it is rare to see any questioning of even the most over-the-top empathic bonding reported within the analytic dyad. Sometimes, these case presentations seem to suggest that the more lost the analyst becomes in the patient's experience, the better, as long as no serious boundary violations occur. I think I have made it clear that there are other reasons to avoid unquestioning and prolonged emotional merger.

D. B. Stern (1988) acknowledged the critical role of empathy, yet also argued that it was not enough.

> To accept an interpersonal view of the analytic relationship demands one to consider and reject the belief that immersion in the patient's world is a reliable route to accurate understanding. One need instead to consider empathically derived knowing as a category of one's reactive experience with and of the patient. (p. 609)

Writing in the same issue of *Contemporary Psychoanalysis*, Moses (1988) argued that too great of an emphasis on empathy, combined with fears of being intrusive, could result in the analyst sitting with "enormous amounts of information" (p. 590) rather than pursing a more active inquiry. He added that this often resulted in the treatment taking place in the analyst's mind rather than in reality.

It is exactly this "sitting with information" I am challenging as an analytic stance. What Stern called the "reactive experience" is the first step in what I am advocating. Case presentations are noticeably lacking in detailed information regarding the analyst's thoughts and feelings in an ongoing way. Negative thoughts and feelings are almost nonexistent in reporting unless they are tied to an enactment.

I think we need to go beyond our passive responding and figure out how to productively use the vast array of internal responses we have to our patients. This will not happen, of course, if we continue to place such heavy emphasis on what we do not know, rather than what we do. I think the fear of doing harm has resulted in a stultifying reliance on emotional merger with the patient, as stated previously, rather than a more active one that necessarily involves some careful experimentation. We cannot cross into a new frontier in analysis without taking chances. If we can overcome our insistence on seeing our patients as fragile infants, I think we could productively engage with them in trying new interventions.

On a related topic, I think we emphasize empathy to the point that there is no expectation of interventions that are not necessarily empathic. For example, I treated a woman for several years who was single, lonely, and in despair about ever meeting a man who would want her. She cried at almost every session, and her tears were real. Yet at the same time, she would eventually get around to displaying self-pity during each session, often with a pronounced whining quality. I often asked myself how I could possibly find a way to let her know that she whined without being cruel and hurtful.

That day finally arrived when, after spending most the session bemoaning her single status, she looked right at me and asked for feedback. She said her friends seemed to tire of hearing about her plight: "Was there something in how she presented herself that turned people off?" I took a deep breath and said that while her pain was very real, she often slipped into self-pity, which most people don't respond well to. I was both relieved and delighted when she said enthusiastically, "Yes, I do whine! I got that from my mother. And I hate it when she does it. I know I do it, but no one ever calls me on it and it is hard to change on my own. But I feel relieved that you mentioned it and I am going to work on changing that." Unsurprisingly, she did. I understand there is no blueprint possible for how or when to make such interventions, but I think we could benefit from talking more about interventions that are constructive and helpful, like behavioral feedback, especially when it is not directly empathic in the moment. (Analytic writers often label all interventions that work as inherently empathic, which I see as too general to be useful.)

The gist of this chapter is congruent with Moses' (1988) statements, in that I have attempted to debunk our over-investment in both the concept of empathy, as well as in the idea that it is automatic and relatively undistorted. I have also argued that empathy, even among trained and dedicated professionals, is easier said than done, and that we need to incorporate the realities of human nature into our theory and practice. We also need a theory of therapeutic action that involves greater participation by the analyst and is congruent with our conception of treatment as a mutual two-person event.

Conclusion

Psychoanalysis has been redefined on many fronts over the past 25 years. Of these changes, perhaps none are more "radical" than the current approach that relies on both neuroscience and early attachment research. To my mind, this necessitates an unsubstantiated generalization of the mother/infant relationship to the adult/adult analytic one, and the equally dubious application of mirror neuron research, as outlined here.

Within this framework, the analyst's primary task is to be the receiver of the patient's emotional communications and to respond empathically. I have made the point here that the direct deposit of the patient's feelings into the analyst's brain is simply not possible, and that empathy itself is a far more complex and challenging issue than we have imagined. Our current views are not supported by the research and they suggest a rather passive and idealized approach to treatment. The continued comparison of the adult patient to an undeveloped infant is equally troubling.

I want to reassert that I am fascinated by neuroscience research and will continue to read and apply it to analytic treatment whenever it is viable to do so, as advocated by Westen and Gabbard (2002). Unfortunately, the research on mirror neurons does not meet the criteria for generalizability to human emotions and intentions, and I must agree with the critics who object to the way it has been implemented in analytic theory and practice.

Note

1 See Hayes (2018): "Learned Matching implies that empathy is both agile and fragile. It can be enhanced and redirected by novel experience, and broken by social change" (p. 499).

References

Alford, C. F. (2016). Mirror neurons, psychoanalysis, and the age of empathy. *International Journal of Applied Psychoanalytic Studies, 13*, 7–23.

Arizmendi, T. G. (2011). Linking mechanisms: Emotional contagion, empathy and imagery. *Psychoanalytic Psychology, 28*, 405–409.

Barrett, L. F. (2017). *How emotions are made: The secret life of the brain.* New York: Houghton Mifflin Harcourt.

Batson, C. D. (1987). Prosocial motivation: Is it ever truly altruistic? *Advances in Experimental Social Psychology, 20*, 65–122.

Batson, C. D. (2009). These things called empathy: Eight related but distinct phenomena. In J. Decety & W. Ickes (Eds.), *The social neuroscience of empathy* (pp. 3–16). Cambridge, MA: Massachusetts Institute of Technology Press.

Bekkali, S., Youssef, G. J., Donaldson, P. H., Albein-Urios, N., Hyde, C., & Enticott, P. G. (2020). Is the putative mirror neuron system associated with empathy? A systematic review and meta-analysis. *Neuropsychology Review.* Retrieved from https://link.springer.com/article/10.1007/s11065-020-09452-6

Blass, R., & Carmeli, Z. (2007). The case against neuropsychoanalysis: On fallacies underlying psychoanalysis' latest scientific trend and its negative impact on psychoanalytic discourse. *International Journal of Psychoanalysis, 88*, 19–40.

Bolding, J. (2019). Criticism regarding the role of the mirror neurons system in empathy yet to be refuted. *Behavior and Neurosciences.* Retrieved from https://fse.studenttheses.ub.rug.nl/19866/1/Scriptie.pdf

Bolognini, S. (1997). Empathy and "empathism." *International Journal of Psychoanalysis, 78*, 279–293.

Bolognini, S. (2001). Empathy and the unconscious. *Psychoanalytic Quarterly, 70*, 447–471.

Boston Change Process Study Group. (2005). The "something more" than interpretation revisited: Sloppiness and co-creativity in the psychoanalytic encounter. *Journal of the American Psychoanalytic Association, 53*, 693–729.

Boston Change Process Study Group. (2018). Moving through and being moved by: Embodiment in development and in the therapeutic relationship. *Contemporary Psychoanalysis, 54*, 299–321.

Brothers, L. (2002). The trouble with neurobiological explanations of mind. *Psychoanalytic Inquiry, 22*, 857–870.

Christov-Moore, L., Simpson, E.A., Coudé, G., Grigaityte, K., Iacoboni, M., & Ferrari, P. F. (2014). *Empathy: Gender effects in brain and behavior. Neuroscience and Biobehavioral Reviews, 46*, 604–627.

Csibra, G. (2004). Mirror neurons and action observation. Is simulation involved? Interdisciplines. http://www.interdisciplines.org/mirror/papers/4

Csibra, G. (2008). Action mirroring and action understanding: an alternative account. In P. Haggard, I. Rosetti, & M. Kawato (Eds.), *Sensorymotor foundations of higher cognition. Attention and performance XXII* (pp. 435–459). London: Oxford University Press.

Damasio, A. R. (2003). *Looking for Spinoza: Joy, sorrow, and the feeling brain*. New York: Harcourt, Inc.

Decety, J. (2010). The neurodevelopment of empathy in humans. *Developmental Neuroscience, 32*, 257–267.

Decety, J., & Lamm, C. (2009). Empathy versus personal distress: Recent evidence from social neuroscience. In J. Decety & W. Ickes (Eds.), *The social neuroscience of empathy* (pp. 199–214). Cambridge, MA: Massachusetts Institute of Technology Press.

Decety, J., & Michalski, K. J. (2010). Neurodevelopmental changes in the circuit underlying empathy and sympathy from childhood to adulthood. *Developmental Science, 13*, 886–899.

Eagle, M., Gallese, V., & Migone, P. (2009). Mirror neurons and mind: Commentary on Vivona. *Journal of the American Psychoanalytic Association, 57*, 559–568.

Engen, H. G., & Singer, T. (2015). Compassion-based emotion regulation up-regulates experienced positive affect and associated neural networks. *Social Cognitive and Affective Neuroscience, 10*(9), DOI: 10.1093/scan/nsv008.

Gallese, V., & Goldman, A. (1998). Mirror neurons and the simulation theory of mind-reading. *Trends in Cognitive Sciences, 2*, 493–501.

Gallese, V., Eagle, M., & Migone, P. (2007). Intentional attunement: Mirror neurons and the neural underpinnings of interpersonal relations. *Journal of the American Psychoanalytic Association, 55*, 131–176.

Goubert, L., Craig, K. D., & Buysse, A. (2009). Perceiving others in pain: Experimental and clinical evidence on the role of empathy. In J. Decety & W. Ickes (Eds.), *The social neuroscience of empathy* (pp. 139–152). Cambridge, MA: Massachusetts Institute of Technology Press.

Hayes, C. (2018). Empathy is not in our genes. *Neuroscience & Biobehavioral Reviews, 95,* 499–507.

Hein, G., & Singer, T. (2008). I feel what you feel but not always: Brain and its modulation. *Current Opinion in Neurobiology, 18,* 153–158.

Herbette, G., & Rimé, B. (2004). Verbalization of emotion in chronic pain patients and their psychological adjustment. *Journal of Health Psychology, 9,* 661–676.

Hickock, G. (2014). *The myth of mirror neurons.* New York: Norton.

Hirsch, I. (2008). *Coasting in the countertransference.* London & New York: Routledge.

Killgore, W.D.S., & Yurgelun-Todd, D. A. (2007). Unconscious process of facial affect in children and adolescents, *Social Neuroscience, 2,* 28–47.

Kim, H., & Han, S. (2018). Does personal distress enhance empathic interaction or block it? *Personality and Individual Differences, 124,* 77–83.

Kohut, H. (1971). *The analysis of the self.* New York: International Universities Press.

Knox, J. (2013). "Feeling for" and "feeling with": Developmental and neuroscientific perspectives on intersubjectivity and empathy. *Journal of Analytical Psychology, 58,* 491–509.

Lamm, C., & Majdandzic, J. (2015). The role of shared neural activation, mirror neurons, and morality in empathy—A critical comment. *Neuroscience Research, 90,* 15–24.

Lanzetta, J. T., & Englis, B. G. (1989). Expectations of cooperation and competition and their effects on observers' vicarious emotional responses. *Journal of Personality and Social Psychology, 56*(4), 543-554. DOI: https://doi.org/10.1037/0022-3514.56.4.543

Manfredi Turillazzi, S. (1994). *Le certezze perdute della psicoanalisi clinica.* Milan: Raffaello Cortina.

McGilchrist, I. (2010). *The master and his emissary: The divided brain and the western world.* New Haven, CT: Yale University Press.

Moses, I. (1988). The misuse of empathy in psychoanalysis. *Contemporary Psychoanalysis, 24,* 577–593.

Pulver, S. E. (2003). On the astonishing clinical irrelevance of neuroscience. *Journal of the American Psychoanalytic Association, 51,* 755–772.

Rizzolatti, G., & Craighero, L. (2004). The mirror-neuron system. *Annual Review of Neuroscience, 27,* 169–192.

Rizzolatti, G., & Sinigaglia, C. (2008). *Mirrors in the brain: How our minds share actions and emotions.* New York: Oxford University Press Inc.

Rothbart, M. K., Ahadi, S. A., & Hershey, K. L. (1994). Temperament and social behavior in childhood. *Merrill Palmer Quarterly, 40,* 21–39.

Schulte-Ruther, M., Markowitsch, H. J., Fink, G. R., & Piefke, M. (2007). Mirror neuron and theory of mind mechanisms involved in face-to-face interactions: A functional magnetic resonance imaging approach to empathy. *Journal of Cognitive Neuroscience, 19,* 1354–1372.

Stern, D. B. (1988). Not misusing empathy. *Contemporary Psychoanalysis, 24,* 596–611.

Stern, D. N. (1985). *The Interpersonal world of the Infant: A view from psychoanalysis and developmental psychology.* New York: Basic Books.

Uithol, S., van Rooij, I., Bekkering, H. & Haselager, P. (2011). What do mirror neurons mirror? *Philosophical Psychology,* 24, 607–623.

Vivona, J. (2006). From developmental metaphor to developmental model" The shrinking role of language in the talking cure. *Journal of the American Psychoanalytic Association,* 54, 877–902.

Vivona, J. M. (2009a). Leaping from brain to mind: A critique of mirror neuron explanations of countertransference. *Journal of the American Psychoanalytic Association,* 57, 525–550.

Vivona, J. M. (2009b). Embodied language in neuroscience and psychoanalysis. *Journal of the American Psychoanalytic Association, 57,* 1327–1360.

Westen, D., & Gabbard, G. O. (2002). Development in cognitive neuroscience: I. Conflict, compromise and connectionism. *Journal of the American Psychoanalytic Association, 50,* 53–98.

Zaki, J., & Ochsner, K. (2012). The neuroscience of empathy: Progress, pitfalls and promise. *Nature Neuroscience, 15,* 675–680.

Zelazo, P. D., Craik, F. I., & Booth, L. (2004). Executive function across the life span. *Acta Psychologica, (Amst), 115,* 167–183.

Chapter 7

Therapeutic action

The only solace we can take in not knowing how psychoanalysis actually works is that those adhering to other therapeutic orientations do not know how treatment works either. This is small consolation and should not deter us from continuing the quest to better understand the essence of therapeutic action. Those of us who are psychoanalysts "know" that our method works because we have seen our patients improve over time, and no one could convince us otherwise. But how do we explain that psychotherapy research seems to indicate that analytic clinicians do not produce results that are superior to other treatments (at least in the short- to medium-term context of most research studies)? The complexity of therapeutic action makes its assessment extraordinarily challenging. The same is true of attempting to generate or augment any theory about how treatment works.

In this chapter, I will examine the issue of therapeutic action from the perspective of our individual and collective psychological contributions to theory and practice. As noted earlier, our theories are personal and reflect our worldviews. I think that our theory, or lack thereof, regarding therapeutic action is no exception. I will discuss the importance of the "match"; review the relevant literature on the efficacy of treatment; discuss our reluctance to claim knowledge or authority; provide a brief overview of analytic theories of therapeutic action; examine the relevant variables contained with the context of therapeutic action; and then elaborate my own stance.

The common thread

For decades, psychoanalysts have been shaking their heads in response to the research that says our outcomes are no better than anyone else's. Given the length and depth of both our theories and our training, how do we understand this? Ackerman and Hilsenroth (2003) confirmed that patients' report of positive outcome was not related to theoretical orientations. Shedler (2010) offers the explanation that many behavioral therapists rely on interventions that are classically psychodynamic, thus blurring the assumed distinctions thought to exist. Furthermore, therapists who do adhere rigidly to manuals and cognitive instructions tend to have poorer outcomes. So perhaps the contributions of more than 100 years of psychoanalysis have had a greater impact on all clinicians than is widely recognized.[1]

But I would also argue that the universal shared early experiences of clinicians explored in this volume crosses theoretical lines, thus accounting for some of these similarities. The research supporting therapists' early experiences as family caregivers is not limited to psychoanalysts. So perhaps we have similar blind spots, similar strengths, and similar ways of behaving with patients because we have a shared perspective on the world, in spite of our differences.

It seems that a behavioral therapist and a psychoanalyst were both highly likely to have been assigned as caretakers to their suffering family members, but because of both innate factors and other life experiences, took different paths to becoming therapists. As a psychoanalyst who has treated many psychotherapists, I have little doubt regarding the clinical significance of personal treatment as it relates to therapy outcome. I believe it is essential for those who engage in deep, long-term work, regardless of theoretical orientation.

But what about the contribution of the patient? I would add that not only do therapists choose their theories and preferred interventions based on personal preferences but also patients have similar preferences that determine who they are comfortable working with. Different therapeutic approaches appeal to different patients—another factor essential to creating a match. The patient who fits with a behaviorist is probably not the same patient who experiences a good fit with a psychoanalyst—especially over time. I believe that not only do clinicians choose their theory based on their early life experiences and innate qualities, but that patients *choose us on similar grounds.* Although my theory is not proven, it is worth considering as a determining factor given that the retention rate in therapy ranges from

30% to 50%. In other words, the match is not occurring with the frequency one would like to see.

If you make the comparison of finding the right therapist to finding the right partner, or even the right friends, it is easy to see why it can require multiple efforts to find the right match. Without sufficient awareness of how the match occurs, it can be unduly discouraging for both analyst and patient when it fails to materialize. Both may spend too much time avoiding the decision to end the relationship, each feeling at fault for the results of the mismatch. Conversely, the patient who leaves quickly because he or she accurately detects that the match is not a good one has made a wise decision on their own behalf. Oftentimes, therapists can fail to make this determination for themselves out of guilt, shame, or self-interest.

During a recent International Association for Relational Psychoanalysis and Psychotherapy (IARPP) online colloquium, I was surprised to hear from analysts across the world that they had been "ghosted" by patients several times. For those not familiar with this term, it means that the patient simply stopped coming, with no subsequent communication, leaving the analyst confused and hurt. Frequently, these patients had been in treatment for a considerable period of time.

An unsatisfying therapy experience is discouraging for both analyst and patient, and it may produce a retreat from further efforts to seek treatment in the short term. But do most patients who do not stay with one therapist end up never getting treatment? I doubt that. Many of my patients have seen several therapists for short to medium lengths of time before seeing me for a longer duration. They didn't stay in their former treatments because they were targeted for symptom relief only, felt there was not a good match between them and their therapists, or benefited from treatment until bumping up against the limitations of the therapist, themselves, or the relationship.

Many treatments seem to be beneficial to a point, then encounter some obstacle to going further. However, this makes sense if you take treatment seriously as a relationship. The terms on which we connect with one person can be very different from the way we connect with another. And, often to our chagrin, all close relationships are ultimately gratifying *and* frustrating. One person cannot hope to provide the avenue to exploring all of our important issues. But the ideal match would provide what was most needed at the time the patient is seeking treatment.

A savvy patient is one who knows what she needs and acts on this intuitive knowledge. And a patient who is difficult to treat for one analyst may have a much easier time with another one. I do not believe this issue can be decided on the basis of diagnosis or personality style. Since every analyst and patient match are unique, it is not possible to determine the match on basis of character organization or symptomology. Also, even our shortcomings (or the patient's) need not be an obstacle to working with someone with whom we can invest. As Crastnopol (2019) says, "It should be noted that with regard to certain flaws, a therapist's objective weakness can mar the work with *one* patient, while still being relatively un-impactful or even functioning as an asset in working with *another*" (p. 406). Similarly, I would add that the *patient's objective weakness can mar the work with one analyst but not another.* I would guess that the reader just blanched a bit at reading this last sentence. Isn't that a negative judgment about a patient? Yes, it is. But no more so than making these judgments about ourselves. Our mutual vulnerability and character flaws simply cannot be omitted from the equation, especially at the outset when a therapeutic alliance is being built. Besides, a patient who stretches the truth may seem like a "liar" to one analyst and more like a "creative storyteller" to another. These individual perceptions make all the difference in establishing a good relationship. And our reluctance to admit that we have these feelings and assessments about each other does not erase their impact.

Also, a patient who is enlivened by and highly responsive to analytic interventions may reject a behavioral approach and vice versa, even if the clinicians are equally empathic, concerned, and genuine. It seems that the potential for therapeutic action might be intimately connected to a shared worldview, even if that shared experience or perspective is not easily observed and takes time to discover. And flaws or weaknesses do not necessarily exclude the possibility of a good match and a successful treatment. The exception to this is the necessity of the analyst demonstrating the aforementioned qualities of empathy, warmth, genuine concern, and commitment. Analysts who are cold, removed, hostile, and/or overly-intellectualized predictably fail to engage productively with their patients.

Characterizing the match

Thus, we begin with these positive analyst characteristics, along with a successful match, as the necessary preconditions for therapeutic action. Without these preconditions, I think it is nearly impossible to meaningfully define therapeutic action. It does not exist as a concept if it has no framework to contain it. Proper consideration of the match, in particular, is crucial to our attempts to assess the success and the mechanism of any treatment. Kantrowitz (1993, 2002) is a pioneer on this topic. She wisely notes that both similarities and differences can be critical factors in the match, both in positive and negative directions.

> Match highlights the similarities and differences between the participants. Similarities may lead to understanding but also to blind spots and defensive collusion. Differences may lead to curiosity and exploration but also failures in empathy and engagement; either may facilitate or impede the process. The effect of the match may change during the course of treatment. Factors that initially benefit engagement in analytic work may later impede it. (2002, p. 347)

Our theories of therapeutic action do not account for the differences related to phases of treatment, nor do they account for the essential role of the match. If you have a bad match, you can follow all manner of good technical advice and solid theory of therapeutic action and still get nowhere. A good theory of therapeutic action, rather than trying to accommodate every type of patient population, should be built on solid principles, address the different phases of treatment, and be predicated on a good match from the start. And, as Kantrowitz points out, what works well in one phase of treatment may not work well in another—an idea that has failed to take hold in the analytic world.

The overemphasis on harmony

We tend to perceive ongoing harmony and good relations between analyst and patient as predicting a positive, therapeutic outcome. With the notable exception of Hirsch (1983), the mother/infant-based blissful relationship receives little scrutiny in the current analytic literature. And too often the natural emergence of negative transference reactions is erroneously labeled as impasse, enactment, or negative therapeutic reaction. As I stated earlier, therapists tend to be conflict-avoidant and too often rush to re-establish harmony rather than allow aggression and conflict to see the light of day. Our tendency to idealize our suffering patients can also result in a failure to explore their sexual and aggressive impulses. Kantrowitz (2002) illustrates this point.

> Neither patients' nor analysts' comfort or discomfort with their engagement is a reliable indicator of analytic benefit. A longitudinal study of analytic outcome showed the match of patient and analyst to be the single factor which illuminated the areas of analytic impasse (Kantrowitz et al., 1989, 1990). Sometimes neither party was aware of the blind spot. Both believed the analyses to be very successful, but comparison of pre- and post-psychological tests showed a major area to be unchanged. For example, their mutual valuation of creativity led to an analyst's interpreting a patient's fantasy of "pouring molten lead" on people as "free expression of fantasy"—and failing to recognize or analyze the aggression. (p. 347)

In line with Kantrowitz's thinking, at the outset of treatment, we need to be thinking not only about how we might be engaged with a prospective patient through empathy and genuine interest but also how we might facilitate the expression of negative emotions and conflict within that treatment, as I outlined in Chapter 4. This position stands in contrast to the current emphasis on "holding" and becoming the new and improved object.

The case of Beth

Beth, a 27-year-old performer, began treatment with the stated issues of loneliness, anxiety, and concerns about her dependency on her mother. She had recently returned to live in Milwaukee, having traveled for some time with a theatre company. During the time she was away, she enjoyed the company of many friends and also dated regularly. Her longest intimate relationship was three years; they broke up after she discovered that her boyfriend had cheated on her. At the same time, the pandemic put a hold on her performing career, so she decided to return to her home town.

Beth presented as attractive, charming, and very funny. She was quite insightful about many of her flaws and described her co-dependent relationship with her mother in hysterically funny vignettes. I found myself laughing throughout the first few sessions—much to her delight. In the past, I thought it necessary for me to stifle this kind of response, thinking it would reinforce her need to entertain others and hide her anxiety and sadness. But over the years, I have learned that when someone's identity revolves around a certain characteristic, like being humorous, it is more rejecting than otherwise not to respond genuinely. If I had not found her amusing, or forced myself not to smile or laugh, I think we would not have been a match.

By the third session, and following a burst of laughter at one of her descriptions, I said to her, "There is no question that you are enormously entertaining, and it certainly is fun to laugh with you. But the scenarios you are describing sound very burdensome and I imagine that these circumstances are quite painful for you." Beth looked a bit surprised, and she fell into silence for a brief time. Then, slowly, tears starting running down her cheeks. As she wept my eyes teared up, which I know she saw.

In the sessions that followed, Beth usually began with some funny story or take on her relations with her family, but then gradually moved toward talking about her fears, guilt, and resentments. As her treatment progressed, she said she had no idea how much pain she was covering up with her humor and began the long struggle of exploring those feelings.

Beth's central issues were her symbiotic relationships with her parents, particularly her mother, and the consequent inability to fall in love and commit to a partner. She also suffers from acute anxiety. I realized that I could quickly establish a warm relationship with Beth. We talked easily and liked each other. But I also reminded myself not to be too enamored of her, or want too much for her, because as strong as she was in many ways, she also has a long road to the independence she craves. Enmeshed her entire life with her parents, she did not realize how this contributed to her not finding a long-lasting relationship, and also to her anxiety when she was not in contact with her family. As these realties sunk in, her sadness increased.

Sometimes, I had to resist the urge to take the edge off her pain, either by failing to go deeper in exploring it or generating humor myself. At one point when she was crying, I felt a strong desire to comfort her. Then I suddenly came up with a humorous comment in my mind. In fact, I almost smiled in response to my internal fantasy. I asked myself "What on earth are you doing?" Clearly this was a defense against her pain, which I was able to successfully manage as I internally worked through what was happening. But I could still feel a certain discombobulation when the session ended.

Beth and I enjoy a close and warm relationship. But I believe we both know that at some point she will resent her dependence on me and the abyss that she painfully inhabits as a result of separating more from her family. I will be identified as the instrument of her pain. And it is vital that I accept that role and not fight to be seen as the "good mother." An essential aspect of my role is that I suffer my own pain at being seen in a negative light, of being "responsible" for her pain, and of feeling the inevitable guilt that accompanies it. I am cognizant of the need to resist reliving my role as family caregiver and soother.

As Beth began her efforts to be more independent of her mother, she was astounded to see that her mother was very cooperative. They had had a heart-to-heart talk, and her mother sincerely wants to do what is best for Beth. When Beth told me about a particular incident when her mother actually nicely refused her offer of assistance, I noted that it seemed her mother loved her enough to try to change. This was very gratifying for Beth, and relieving. Beth does not want me to criticize her mother or dethrone her. She wants me to constructively address their over-involvement, noting what works and is gratifying in their relationship as well as what doesn't. By taking this position, I allay Beth's fears about having to give her mother up. As a result, she is also freed from thinking she must choose between us.

Interestingly, Loewald's (1960) conception of therapeutic action implies a displacing of the mother to make room for the introjected analyst. Should Beth just realize how her mother failed her, allowing me to become the superior mother that she can identify with instead? I realize that Loewald was not intending any slur against mothers, but nonetheless, in the reality of treatment, his proposition promotes the aforementioned ideal of the analyst's superiority. It also conveys a level of disrespect for many well-meaning yet deeply flawed mothers.

Beth's worst fear is losing her mother. Either she will be abandoned by her mother, wish to break the attachment herself, or some combination of the two. In either event, she experiences existential anxiety at the loss of an overwhelming attachment that has defined her, and she feels equally anxious at the thought of becoming her own person, which she equates with being alone in the world. She also feels tremendous guilt at the thought of being separate from her mother and no longer accommodating her needs. (I think this primal fear of loss was poignantly depicted in the novel and film, *The English Patient*.)

Although not all patients feel this way, of course, I find it more common than not for family ties and loyalty to be a significant obstacle to individual growth. And this developmental reality, so aptly noted by Feiner and Levenson (1968–69), Mitchell (1988), Searles (1973), and others, is profound. We adapted to our parents out of the primal fear of losing them, which never leaves us. Our loyalties are not just to our authentic selves but also to them. As Mitchell (1988) said, "Operating with old illusions and stereotyped patterns reduces anxiety and provides security not simply because the illusions and patterns are *familiar*, but also because they are *familial* and preserve a sense of loyalty and connection" (p. 291).

Beth finds losing her mother indistinguishable from losing herself. The less I do to stoke that anxiety, the better. My job is not to be a better mother or better person. My job is to help Beth better observe, understand, and feel the enmeshment with her mother. She is open to changing her behavior and has begun asserting herself in small ways. She is also becoming painfully aware of how she will lure her mother back into their co-dependent rhythms if her mother backs away.

Facilitating Beth's insight, particularly her participation in the symbiotic family dynamics, represents as aspect of therapeutic action. Beth's parents have each, in their own way, begun making small steps toward being more independent of each other and of her. Beth is astounded by this and was able to observe herself offering to do things for them to re-establish their overreliance on her. She also cried profusely when she told me this. She is struggling mightily with her desire to change and become her own person, yet also must deal with the fear and emptiness that temporarily fill the void left by even small steps toward separation.

The reader may ask how this is different than any other analytic approach to treatment. My answer is that, of course, what I say to patients and what I emphasize in my own conceptualizations cannot be vastly different than what others do. One of the points I am fond of making is that human nature cannot be transcended and that our repertoires are necessarily limited by this and by other factors in our lives. So it is really more about the match, the accuracy of my perceptions regarding what the patient needs, and my ability to facilitate that movement.

I can honestly say that my treatments have been shorter and more successful as I have gained confidence in being candid with patients, educating them about the process, letting them know what I am observing, and respecting their strengths as well as acknowledging their deficits. I had only been treating Beth for a few weeks when we began the process of self-awareness described here. I could have easily spent months or longer simply being sympathetic and providing a holding environment for her. And, granted, some patients do need this. But Beth didn't, and I was quick to recognize her capacity to manage both the realities of her situation and her intense feelings.

My basic rejection of the "developmental tilt" approach, while still focusing on important attachment issues, empowers me and my patients. I do not view my patients as children, even when we are focused on the pain that emanates from their early experiences. More importantly, I fear that our current central focus on trauma plays to not only our patients' weaknesses but also to our own. Does the popularity of victim status stimulate our own rescue fantasies and encourage us to engage in an ill-fated attempt at mutual healing rather than self-awareness and integration? And does it fail to meet the standard of respect for our adult patients' present developmental status and demonstrated resilience?

From the very first session, I actively look for the patient's strengths, make sure I include them whenever I am giving feedback, and try to imagine what a good outcome would look like. I then think about how what actions on my part would best facilitate that outcome. All of this occurs in the context of what the patient is seeking, of course, and includes conversations about the agreed upon goals that are the mark of a successful treatment.

As Kantrowitz said, my role in the beginning of treatment, though still based on a strong relationship with Beth, necessarily shifts from soothing presence to facilitator of interpsychic and interpersonal conflict. Different phases of treatment evolve within the context of a strong analyst/patient bond, challenging the analyst to rise to the occasion. And I would add that acting as a facilitator of strong emotion, particularly grief, represents a critical aspect of the analyst's role in therapeutic action. I believe that infusing the analytic sessions with emotion, *as a deliberate action*, serves us better than defining therapeutic action as a series of enactments. But before continuing with my own views, I would like to outline and comment on the views expressed by others.

A brief history of therapeutic action

Donnel Stern (1996), in his classic piece on therapeutic action, notes that historical transition from the interpretive model, defined by the analyst and patient being two separate individuals, with analyst as interpreter of the patient's experience. The patient's suffering was determined by his or her internal conflicts, which were identified and clarified by the analyst. Gradually, this model was expanded by developmental models focusing on the patient's experience of being known and understood. Stern points out that

> Psychoanalysis, then, as more and more frequently portrayed as a process of maturation, a matter of resuming arrested development through an attachment to a benign parental figure who offers a kind of experience that may actually be new but is at the very least the necessary condition for change. (p. 278)

But Stern also notes that the analyst who focuses on developmental lags and offers the patient a new and presumably safer environment in which to grow is never off the hook for making decisions about what is true. For example, when the patient criticizes us, we must decide to some extent whether or not that criticism is true. If we apologize when we do not really believe we did anything wrong, we are setting up an inauthentic relationship and possibly short-circuiting the patient's attempt to be in conflict with us. If we have said or done something that is objectively insensitive or hurtful, then an apology of some sort is probably in order. However, making this determination is easier said than done.

Black (2003) illustrates a case when she and the patient are at odds over an incident in a session. A serious conflict ensues, which she deems an enactment. It is not truly resolved, but Black stands by her decision not to placate the patient with surrendering her own version of events in favor of the patient's. She refuses the invitation to issue a false mea culpa. Black readily admits that she may be blind to something that took place, but she cannot honestly share the patient's view of what happened, no matter how hard she tries. I was relieved to see Black's willingness to publicly admit that when there is a "reality dispute," the analyst cannot merely capitulate. Authenticity trumps confirming the patient's reality, even if the analyst is unaware of some contributing factor.

I think her case report illustrates that even if the analyst cannot, and should not, be the arbiter of truth, neither can she be the unwitting sacrificial lamb for the purpose of shoring up the patient. Had Black been willing to subsume her will to the patient's, I believe the result would have been nontherapeutic. I have found that people always know when they are being placated, and while they may experience some triumph in the moment, they ultimately feel disappointed and disrespected. To my mind, authenticity is a critical variable in therapeutic action.

Frank and Bernstein (2012) discuss the evolution of our theories of therapeutic action, noting that our defined role has shifted from providing "precise" interpretations to providing a new relational experience. They say this new relationship constitutes "the crucible of change" (p. 3) in contemporary psychoanalysis. Although I agree that the current focus on the new relational experience is significantly different from older analytic models of therapeutic action, it also shares some distinct qualities. First and foremost is the proposition that the analyst is front and center, offering up both a model for affective regulation and one that might be internalized by the patient. This can be seen in the classic and oft-cited articles on therapeutic action by Strachey (1934) and Loewald (1960).

Though rooted in the precise interpretation period outlined by Frank and Bernstein, their conceptualizations of therapeutic action rely heavily on the analyst as internalizable, good object. Strachey (1934) is a bit more conservative on this issue, warning against actually trying to be either "good" or "bad" in reality. Rather, he emphasized interpretive technique, saying that the analyst's ongoing "mutative interpretations" gradually allow the patient to discover the true nature of the analyst (the external object), resulting in a more realistic view of the analyst, himself, and the world. Yet, internalization of the analyst remains a prominent feature of his theory.

Loewald (1960), on the other hand, believes the analyst serves as a new object that is significantly better than the patient's parents. Again, while seeming to promote neutrality, the objective is for the analyst to truly be the new, good object who is introjected by the patient. Through "scrupulous neutrality" and "objectivity," the analyst facilitates the therapeutic process through interpretation. He likens the patient's incremental introjections of the analyst to the gradual internalization of the mother during childhood.

Both Strachey and Loewald, albeit in slightly different terms, hold the analyst up as a linchpin of therapeutic action. I do want to acknowledge that this discussion is based on a snapshot of their much more complex and erudite explorations of therapeutic action. I am deliberately focusing in these singular, yet critical, aspects of their theories for the purposes of my thesis. My implied suggestion is that analysts have held themselves up as paragons of mental health for generations. Loewald actually goes a bit further by comparing himself to a sculptor, who carves away not stone, but the patient's neurotic distortions.

Questioning the focus on the analyst

In spite of their significant contributions to our thinking about therapeutic actions, Strachey's and Loewald's views reflect a tradition that places the analyst securely "above" the patient's world. I find that virtually all theories of therapeutic action elevate the analyst's role and character above the patient's. Even in this era of acknowledged mutuality in the analytic dyad, the patient's role, responsibilities, and character take a back seat to the analyst's. Ironically, at the same time the analyst assumes this superior position, the patient's weaknesses and limitations remain neglected. For example, I cannot recall the last time I heard anyone use the word "prognosis." As Rangell (1992) notes,

> There are patients who change from the very beginning, patients who show no evidence or inclination to change near or even at the end, some who change after the analysis (from unconscious readiness only then), and some who never do. Some change, for the worse. (p. 419)

I agree with him and think we could benefit from more discussion about this, rather than assuming that if the analyst is just "good enough," he or she can provide a transformative experience for most, if not all, of those who come for treatment. For example, my patient Beth is obviously psychologically minded, intelligent, young, and seeking change. She is not typical of most patients, exhibiting unusual resilience and tolerance for painful insights.

The reader is unlikely to be surprised by my taking exception to the analyst as new good object—particularly as this applies to therapeutic action. Do our patients really improve because we are better people than their parents were? Also, is it not disingenuous, from Loewald to present-day attachment frameworks, to argue for a mother–infant developmental model *at the same time we are lamenting the pervasive failures of mothering?* This makes no sense to me. Are we not prone to the same failures of empathy, disinterest, self-interest, and distractions as were our patients' mothers?

Granted, we are not burdened with the stress of caring for them 24-7. We have the luxury of limited contact with our patients; a level of psychological sophistication not achieved by many; and a volitional engagement marked by professional interest and gratification. But that still falls far short of us being better people. In fact, I would argue that this injunction to be "better people" has contributed heavily to our unrealistic pursuit of perfection and equally led to us feeling like frauds and failures. One also has to question the moralism inherent in implying that our patients and/or their mothers are inferior to us. Whether we use those labels or not, that is the implication. Again, to what extent have we replaced "superior knowledge" from the days when we thought we knew everything, with being "superior mothers" who fill the developmental void left by inadequate parenting or trauma?

Why do we need to be better anyway? I think we should settle for being different—offering the services of a trained professional who can facilitate insight and emotion regulation. What do we realistically offer our patients that helps them to change? I think what most distinguishes us from other people in our patients' lives is our ability to understand what interventions might be helpful and then to execute them. This occurs within the aforementioned context of genuine concern, but it is not based on our capacity for unconditional love. Granted, we do come to love many of our patients to varying degrees. But I have been successful in treating difficult people whom I was dedicated to treating but did not love.

I think it is easy to fall into responding out of our patients unrealistic, but understandable, wishes for a better mothering experience. It can be heartbreaking to listen to their poignant wish to be rescued—to have the pains of their childhood experiences erased. But do they really want us to dethrone their mothers and replace them with us? Is that concept more about their needs or more about our own? And what part does our own early experience contribute to our desire to both "have and be" the good mother? Finally, with the understanding that some introjection occurs in any long-term relationship, are we failing to prioritize the patient's active pursuit of his own secure identity over internalizing the analyst?

Although I appreciate that the patient's ability to recognize the feelings and thoughts of others is crucial to healthy functioning, do we not overvalue the patient's ability to "mentalize" us, particularly if they are not having a significant problem with recognizing others? When is this more about our narcissistic needs rather than the patient's growth and development? I find that some patients have little interest in figuring me out, having entered treatment with the objective of resolving internal conflicts. My feelings do not come into play for them unless they somehow disrupt the equilibrium they have come to expect. I sometimes wonder if our strong interest in the patient's impressions of us has replaced the erotic transference as a major source of gratification.

It has been well stablished that the heart of therapeutic change is the relationship. Yet, we do not know *what is therapeutic* in the relationship. If it is primarily being caring and accepting, couldn't a close social relationship provide that better than we can? I think that the analyst as a new object has merit, but not in the way we think about it. I think is has more do with the unique characteristics of the therapeutic relationship, as well as the unique setting provided in treatment. Naturally, my longstanding efforts to identify affective experience as critical to therapeutic action are a given in my view of what is efficacious in treatment.

As patients often say themselves, the experience of focused attention on what they are thinking and feeling for an hour or more per week is an amazing experience. And while they may also balk at the asymmetry, it provides a degree of unilateral focus on them that cannot be replicated elsewhere. Having this opportunity to dig deep into feelings, have the space to self-reflect and integrate—all in the presence of an empathic and concerned other—constitutes a kind of "hot house" relationship that is truly unique. I think we have not sufficiently credited the treatment environment itself for promoting the sense of safety, space, and time for self-examination. That is why boundaries remain a cornerstone of the therapeutic environment.

Throughout this chapter, I am working to identify the essential elements of therapeutic action. I will also continue to identify what I believe to be conceptualizations that likely detract from therapeutic success. At the same time, I want to acknowledge the inevitable obstacles to creating any comprehensive notion of therapeutic action. Aron (2000) wisely said in his paper on self-reflexivity that "Understanding the therapeutic action of psychoanalysis is therefore one of the 'big' topics, beyond the scope of any single article" (p. 668)—or any book chapter, of course. I am also inclined to agree with Friedman (2008). Though skeptical regarding the possibility of any agreed upon account of what constitutes psychoanalysis, he said, "Nevertheless, we must keep trying to capture the specialness of analytic treatment or else give up all claims to a procedure" (p. 437). In that vein, I feel compelled to make an attempt at elucidating my thoughts on this undeniably complex and difficult issue.

Contemporary issues in therapeutic action

Having illustrated how important the match is to a successful treatment, I want to selectively review some recent literature on therapeutic action.[2]

Gabbard and Westen (2003), in their incisive article on therapeutic action, note that the delineation between interpretative and relational aspects of therapeutic action no longer exists. It is generally accepted that they are intertwined and are used as indicated with individual patients. Furthermore, there is widespread acceptance that the therapeutic process occurs at all levels of consciousness. I believe our agreement on these issues goes a long way toward a theory of therapeutic action, were it not for our reluctance to discuss and implement techniques that derive directly from these theoretical propositions.

Gabbard and Westen discuss this reluctance to tie any theory of therapeutic action to actual techniques. They quote Mitchell (1997) on the impossibility of developing techniques because each treatment requires a "custom designed" approach. I find myself simultaneously agreeing and disagreeing with this idea. I firmly believe that a large part of the initial therapeutic process involves becoming acquainted with the patient—trying out different interventions and seeing what works and what doesn't. Figuring out a rhythm, a mode of being with each other, both in silence and in speech, is equally important.

For example, some very quiet patients want me to match them and be more reserved and tempered in my language. Other quiet patients want me to complement them by saying things they wouldn't and being more spontaneous and gregarious. To me, the only technical aspect of this phenomenon is the one of listening to, and watching for, the patients' responses to how I behave. The principal at work is proper attention to the patient's response at a given point in time, which is inherently "customized," yet also a generalizable proposition across patients.

Some patients clearly do better when their intellects are engaged frequently, whereas others are laser-focused on the relational aspects of the dyad. So Mitchell's notions of "customizing" the treatment fits with being responsive to these individual patient characteristics, which most clinicians do. Part of my educating the patient about the process is telling them that I have to get to know them and understand what is most helpful to them. I doubt that anyone would dispute the value of this perspective.

On the other hand, I cannot endorse the proposition that our clinical decisions result primarily from individualizing treatment. I think we can rely on the consistent application of some basic principles across patients, such as the prime importance of affect, the need for behavioral feedback, the usefulness of deep interpretation, the willingness to confront the patient with distortions and contradictions in values and behaviors, and so on. Psychotherapy research (Ackerman & Hilsenroth, 2003,Barnicot et al., 2014) has confirmed the effectiveness of discussing the process of therapy, agreeing on treatment goals, and talking frankly about the hard work required of the patient, yet the psychoanalytic literature steadfastly eschews such practicality. Emotional honesty and authenticity are also guiding standards for me, though I am aware that none of us can live up to the standard of candor and self-awareness implied by this statement.

I believe that all clinicians have established in their own minds, through a series of successes and failures, which interventions tend to work and which do not. Admittedly, this will be somewhat idiosyncratic. But I think we would not be surprised at our commonality if, instead of guarding what we actually do and say, we were more forthcoming with each other. The adherence to currently accepted views of analytic treatment, combined with the lack of transparency in public presentations, make it impossible for us to collect the experiential data we need to make better decisions about efficacy. Smith (2007) addresses this issue:

> My impression is that the techniques of one analyst that prove useful frequently have much in common with the techniques of another, even though the two analysts may hold different theories of mind; and successful interventions can often be justified after the fact from any number of different theoretical points of view. I should think that a determination of what is therapeutic in analysis might usefully begin with the study of what analysts do and the effects of what they do, leaving aside, for the moment, the theories of mind, pathogenesis, and technique that they adopt (often in retrospect) to explain what they do (or did). (p. 1739)

Without offering any opinions on why we avoid technique, Gabbard and Westen (2003) also agree that we could benefit from moving past our reluctance to speak more openly about what we do. They argue for a more focused approach to therapeutic action, leaving room for multiple theories, with an eye toward systematic strategies at the same time. In their umbrella approach, they say, "A theory of therapeutic action must describe both *what changes* (aim of treatment) and *what strategies* are likely to be useful in facilitating those changes (techniques)" (p. 826).

I couldn't be more in agreement with their statement. They review the literature, including appropriate neuroscience findings, confirming that regardless of theory, most goals "can be understood in terms of altering unconscious associational networks" (p. 828). Some might say this is an updated version of Freud's "making the unconscious conscious," but it goes much further into the details of affect management and regulation. Incorporating significant neuroscience findings, they say, "lasting change requires a *relative* deactivation of problematic links in activated networks and increased activation of new, more adaptive connections, so that the patient will tend to find new, more adaptive compromise solutions" (p. 829).

This statement certainly fits with what most analysts see as an essential aspect of therapeutic action—bringing emotions into awareness and working them through. Emotion is rightly the currency in recent discussions of what brings about change. Gabbard and Westen proceed to review the elements of change currently proposed by analysts, including free association, several categories of interpretation, the impact of the relationship (including modeling), confrontation, exposure, and self-disclosure. They conclude by saying there is no single path to change, although some principles of change are likely to be effective across patients, while others are effective with only a select group.

They also suggest that it would behoove us to focus more on how our multiple strategies interact with each other in actual clinical work and attempt to explicate this in more detail in our case reports. Clearly, my views are very compatible with theirs, particularly the practical notion of discovering what works, both across patients and selectively with certain types of patients. Their view is very much in accord with earlier statements by Safran (2003), who discussed the research paradigm appropriate for a study of therapeutic action: "The *events paradigm* stipulates that rather than attempting to demonstrate that one therapy is more effective than another, we should be studying specific moments in therapy, or events that are critical to change" (p. 451).

Finding out what the patient needs and responding accordingly, whether that be deep empathy, confrontation, education, interpretation, or behavioral feedback, produces positive results. The match naturally includes compatibility between what the patient needs and what the analyst is willing and/or able to provide. Some therapists find constant boundary setting and confrontation to be too arduous and exhausting. Others lose patience with prolonged "walking on egg shells" with a fragile patient. As mentioned previously, what we have to offer can vary based on our personalities, our training, our preferred ways of relating, and our life circumstances.

The reader may recall my earlier example about the patient who began her first session with me following the death of my father. I was atypically both threatened and angered by her derisive comments about my office and my fee, deciding immediately not to treat her. Yet she did see another therapist who she did not immediately criticize and did well with her. So I want to echo Smith's comments about the need for careful study of what we specifically do and say with our patients, but also add our thoughts about how our idiosyncrasies and current life circumstances impact our capacities.

The Boston Change Process Study Group

Those of you who know my work are aware that I have been writing about emotion in analysis since my first book on countertransference (Maroda, 1991). I have been pleased to see how our transition from classical analysis to relational analysis has produced the conclusion that it is the emotion-producing aspects of the relationship that hold the greatest potential for change. Arguably, the most influential proponent of the critical role of emotion in treatment is the Boston Change Process Study Group (BCPSG).

Let me begin by reiterating that Daniel Stern's paradigm-shifting classic *The Interpersonal World of the Infant* (1985) deeply influenced my own work. His research on affective attunement helped me to see some of my dysregulated patients in a whole new light. Although I was never inclined to see my adult patients as infants, I certainly appreciated Stern's explanations for how emotional dysregulation emanates from a dysregulated mother–infant experience.

His ideas about how the mother ideally responds to her maturing infant, especially how she brings her own emotions into play in the back-and-forth rhythms of their ongoing communication, inspired me to think about how to utilize this principle in adult-to-adult interactions. Schore's (1994) groundbreaking application of neuroscience to the psychotherapeutic process was equally influential. Thus was born my own theory of using unfettered facial expressions and self-disclosure to complete the cycle of affective communication, a topic I outlined in detail in my previous work (Maroda, 1999, 2010).

The subsequent writings of the BCPSG clearly resonated deeply with analysts who instinctively knew that emotion was at the heart of therapeutic action. Arguably, saying this out loud was not popular prior to the BCPSG's landmark publication that freed up clinicians to do "something more" than interpretation (Stern et al., 1998). They described therapeutic action as hinging on the success or failure of emotionally connecting with patients. They did not devalue interpretation, but rather expressed their view that these emotional "moments of meeting" needed to be explored and understood.

Unfortunately, they then proceeded to outline their application of neuroscience and implicit communication, defining moments of meeting as the "event that rearranges *implicit relational knowing* for patient and analyst alike" (p. 906). They based these statements on the aforementioned application of mother-infant research and mirror neuron research, which has been criticized widely in the literature. And as Vivona (2006) and others have said, it relies too heavily on unconscious communication rather than deliberate procedures.

From my own perspective, their work emerged during a period when the two-person approach had taken hold and analysts were becoming increasingly aware of the importance of affective commination within the dyad. Hungry for someone to endorse this reality, the BCPSG came into prominence, giving clinicians permission to value and facilitate authentic, emotional moments in treatment. Calling this the "shared implicit relationship" (1998, p. 910), they took a turn that was in direct opposition to my own beliefs and writing. Describing the emotional communication between analyst and patient, they said, "It is a process that is conducted out of awareness most of the time" (p. 910).

Again, this went counter to everything I was reading in the neuroscience literature and experimenting with in my own practice. As the BCPSG (2007, 2018a, 2018b) were creating a whole new vocabulary that, to my mind, emphasized vagueness—for example, "now moments,"

"moments of meeting," "implicit relational knowing," "emergent properties," "moving along," "open space," and "charged other,"—I was focusing on the impact of deliberate self-disclosure, rooted in the analyst's emotional response to the patient. I decided to dig deeper into the mirror neuron research and the attachment research in an attempt to determine the validity of their views versus my own. We were both immersed in attachment and neuroscience, yet coming up with mostly different conclusions about how to incorporate this research into treatment.

The more I read, the more I disagreed with the BCPSG. I think I adequately outlined my issues with their application of mirror neuron research in the previous chapter. I also disagree that the therapeutic action of psychoanalysis resides chiefly in enactment—as stated in Chapter 4. I am also influenced by the affect research that says strong emotions, especially negative ones, are rarely out of awareness over time (Panksepp, 1994).

Suffice it to say that I am not the only critic of the BCPSG's conclusions. Modell (2008) has also criticized them regarding their application of neuroscience. I have already cited Vivona (2009) regarding her differences regarding infant and brain research, as well as the BCPSG's diminution of the importance of verbal communication. Allison and Fonagy (2016) agree, saying verbal communication "provides the backbone of the therapeutic encounter" (p. 284). Ellman and Moskowitz (2008) outline several issues they have with the work of the BCPSG, including what they see as their overreliance on comparing mother–infant interaction to adult treatment, lack of research support for their conclusions, and even their definition of enactment as implicit. On this latter subject, they say,

> [H]aving edited a book on enactments (Ellman & Moskowitz, 1998), which includes chapters by most of the prominent authors in the area, we believe that not one of them viewed enactments as being implicit. This is an example of the BCPSG using a confident tone to move the reader into accepting its unsupported assertions. (pp. 816–817)

I think it is important that our pronouncements be as rooted in research as possible, especially if we are presenting them on that basis.

For the most part, analytic writers are not put to this test because our views are not researched-based, but rather the outgrowth of our reading, our clinical experience, and our imagination. Making scientific claims that cannot be supported leaves the writer more vulnerable to unfavorable critique.

For myself, the idea that the analytic relationship is determined and played out on an unconscious-to-unconscious basis strikes me as highly non-analytic as well as implausible. How do patients gain mastery of their affective worlds without being able to feel, name, and manage their emotions, as Krystal (1988) so elegantly explicated? And how do analysts model these affect regulation skills if they rely on enactment to tell them what they feel? I agree with Vivona (2006, 2019) that we cannot ignore the fact that psychoanalysis takes place through language, in spite of the important impact of presymbolic events in the patient's life. The expression of intrapsychic and interpersonal conflicts is communicated verbally, in spite of the reality of body language. Our facial expressions and posture certainly convey emotion, but not in a manner that can be elucidated in analytic treatment. The analyst's observation of the patient's posture, vocal tone, or facial expressions is, by definition, a verbal event. The patient's exploration of the meaning of those feelings is likewise, by definition, a verbal event.

More recently, the BCPSG (2018a) expands on their thesis in a more recent publication venturing into the world of emotional meeting: "Being moved by another or moving *through* another conveys the dual sense of being moved in feeling and also of transcending space and body boundaries by directly experiencing the other's affective and intention and action orientation toward the world" (p. 303). I understand the appeal of such poetic and philosophical musings about what we do for a living. But if this is what heals people, why don't lovers heal each other? You might argue that to some extent they do, and I would agree. In fact, the BCPSG (2018b) acknowledges the therapeutic potential aspect of close relationships as they outline their concept of "the charged other." But does abstracting and romanticizing our therapeutic roles really serve us or our patients? In the aforementioned paper, the BCPSG make the case for emotional engagement, which is very much in line with my own thinking. It is taking that engagement to increasingly diffuse and undefinable levels that I find unhelpful.

I also find it interesting that the case examples they use in both of these 2018 papers are firmly situated in conscious, verbal exchanges between analyst and patient—primarily relying on the analyst's ability to use humor, generating mutual recognition and laughter. Although in both cases the analyst relied on long-time experience and engagement with their patients, they were not enactments. They were deliberate interventions made by the both analysts, based on their accumulated experience with each patient. Does this not contradict their foundational belief that therapeutic action is rooted in implicit (unconscious) communication? The analysts in these examples did not rely on enactments. One could argue that their interventions were based on knowledge gained through unconscious processes, but is this not true of most human interactions? The stuff of therapeutic action is what we do with what we know, regardless of the source of that knowledge.

How "not-knowing" impacts our efforts to define analytic process

Just as we are prone to avoiding conflict within the analyst dyad, we avoid conflict with our peers. But just as I endorse constructive conflict in treatment, I believe psychoanalysis could benefit from it as well. I agree with Blass (2003, 2010) that it is time for us to express our opinions more emphatically so that we can work toward some kind of consensus about what works and what does not. Not knowing has become a caricature of healthy self-scrutiny and openness. Rather than an expression of acceptance, those who embrace not knowing hold those possessing strong opinions in contempt. Kravis (2013) weighs in on this as follows.

> The warranted suspicion of claims to authoritative knowledge can glibly morph into the unwarranted suspicion of all knowledge claims. As a result, the loss of authoritative knowledge has been accompanied in some quarters by an insidious trashing of what we *do* know. (p. 103)

I think our writing in general lacks specificity regarding our interventions and generally lacks strong convictions. In earlier chapters,

I addressed our fears of being wrong, of being criticized, and of being in conflict with other group members. We save our criticism for "others," seemingly working to preserve our agreed upon narratives, even to the extent of claiming "not knowing" as a preferred position. Seeing more value in respectful differences of opinion, Blass (2010) bemoans our postmodern fear that critiquing current approaches will be viewed as an attack. Arguing for "politically incorrect" acts of declaring our truths, she says,

> [I]t becomes clear that what is needed to critically examine analytic theories is a process of reflection and dialogue. While this process cannot provide certain proof regarding the truth of a theory, what it can provide is a deeper and more precise understanding of one's own theory and those of others. Misperceptions can be put aside, fundamental differences recognized, and the true grounds of our thinking brought to the fore. (p. 60)

She joins Gabbard and Westen, Fonagy, Jacobs, Mills, myself, and others in this call to greater examination of our work and the strength of our convictions. A good example of these efforts is Roy Barsness's (2018) study of "core competencies," where his qualitative research revealed what experienced relational analysts did during a typical day with patients. He also asked them to note what ideals and principals guided their interventions. Cornelius (2018) provides research evidence for the efficacy of analytic treatment as compared to other modalities, including psychopharmacology, in that same volume. Blaglys and Hilsenroth (2000) and Diener et al. (2007) all confirmed the importance of affective experience.

Although the original intent of the founders of the two-person movement was reducing the authoritarianism and arrogance often associated with classical analysis, I believe we have over-corrected in this regard. Benjamin (1997) said, "As valuable as we have found the stance of tolerating not-knowing and the reflection on uncertainty, it is unquestionably dangerous to move from that stance into an ideal of not-knowing" (p. 797). More than 20 years later, I think we have moved into just such a position. In that light, I invite the reader to examine my own theoretical constructs with skepticism and an eye toward their own experience and point of view.

What therapist attitudes are helpful?

The question we have failed to answer is, "What occurs within the context of the relationship that is therapeutic?" I use the word "therapeutic" with the intended meaning of reducing the patient's symptoms as well as facilitating emotional regulation, self-awareness, and self-control. I think the argument about insight versus symptom relief has been safely put to rest and need not be addressed here. Our patients want both, and we wish to facilitate both.

First and foremost, I think it is time to reconceptualize the analytic relationship as one of adult to adult. Doing so would not require us to relinquish our attachment-informed perspective. But it would necessitate jettisoning unfailing commitment to caretaking and protective avoidance of negative feelings. It would require us to admit more candidly to both our strengths and weaknesses, as well as our patients'. It seems that since rejecting the use of diagnosis as too pejorative, we have replaced it with viewing our patients as abused and traumatized children. Rather than being a passing fad, the clinical focus on our patients' inner damaged infant/child seems to be increasing. As stated previously, I think this represents a distortion of the impact and mechanism of emotional engagement and therapeutic alliance.

The reason this concerns me so much is because I think that the clinician who values truth and authenticity, no matter how difficult these may be to discern, behaves differently than the clinician who wants to heal the wounds of the patient's past through their sacrifice and unconditional caring. Interestingly, a study of the impact of clinician behaviors on client depression revealed that "Clinician unconditional regard seems quite distinct in that it was not associated with outcome, and was only weakly correlated with the other subscales" (Barnicot et al., 2014, p. 115).

You may ask how these ideas fit with the aforementioned need for empathy, caring, and concern for forming a therapeutic alliance. I believe the answer lies in the point made by Gabbard and Westen (2003) regarding the neglected aspect of phase-specific behaviors. Early in treatment, the patient is seeking understanding and signs that the therapist is sympathetic to the painful situations they bring to treatment. They are not looking for deep interpretations or confrontations. But, as Hirsch (2008) has said, we need a statute of limitations on this holding and nurturing behavior. To assume that this is what our patients need and want over time anchors them in the infant position. Lingiardi et al. (2018), in their review of studies of psychodynamic therapist characteristics and positive outcome, report that "facilitative interpersonal skills (such as verbal fluency, emotional expression, warmth or positive regard, and empathy) predicted better outcomes in short-term therapies … whereas in longer term therapies, this effect was very weak" (p. 97).

This research suggests that once an atmosphere of empathy and safety has been established, it no longer needs to be the primary focus of treatment. Once our patients trust us and begin to surrender to their emotional experiences, what they need from us evolves. They begin to ask or note how we feel in response to them. They want to know what we think of them, and they want us to use our intellects and experience to facilitate greater insight and awareness. They also want us to acknowledge their flaws and missteps, which we too often equate with being rejecting and punitive. I have repeatedly said, and continue to believe, that feedback given in a non-punitive, matter-of-fact matter is greatly therapeutic and greatly appreciated. For example, when a long-time patient asks me directly if he or she "was a pain in the ass last time we met?" and I agree that they were, I will simply say, "Yes, actually you were." This type of encounter is almost always followed by a shared smile or laugh, then by a discussion of what feelings or circumstances led to the regretted behavior. Sometimes, the behavior was related to something I had said or done, but just as often it has to do with the patient's intrapsychic conflicts or events outside the treatment.

As stated earlier in this volume, idealized views of either patient or analyst are based on the mutual desire to be rescued that ultimately derails the analytic process. Not accepting our patients' realistic views of themselves fails the test of anything approaching true acceptance. Do our attempts at unconditional acceptance not only deny the inevitable negative feelings we sometimes have toward our patients, but also communicate our need to see our patients as innocents? Since they know that no one can rightly claim this status, they are left with needing to hide their darkest sides from us. In doing so, they protect themselves from our denial—a denial that is not only about their darker sides but also about our own.

I want to add some particular notes on the treatment of those who were traumatized as children. The treatment of trauma, increasingly more broadly defined, has arguably become the bread and butter of contemporary analytic writing. Along with this prominence, I have observed that, as part of the tendency for clinicians to infantilize these patients, they create special circumstances for treating them that break down our earlier conceptions of acceptable boundaries, idealize their suffering, and deny their individual flaws and negative behaviors.

Our patients come to treatment for self-knowledge and self-acceptance. If we persist in idealizing their suffering, and their responses to that suffering, we will fail to identify sources of guilt and shame. Granted, some of these feelings are unwarranted, particularly in as much as they emerge from childhood trauma—particularly sexual abuse. And I appreciate our role in reducing sadistic superego assaults. Yet we must also leave room for reality-based observations of failings, character flaws, and bad behavior. Excusing the patients "sins," for lack of a better word, does not facilitate self-acceptance. I think forgiveness facilitates self-acceptance. Minimizing or denying the patients self-identified regrettable actions supports the idea that such actions or feelings make them bad people.

A basic outline of therapeutic action

Time and space limitations do not permit any detailed discussion of techniques in this chapter, but I refer the reader to my previous work (Maroda, 1991, 1999, 2010) where I do provide detailed examples of self-disclosure and other affect-oriented interventions, along with suggested guidelines for their use. For my purposes here, I will simply describe the basic elements of therapeutic action, aimed at integrating the different ideas presented in this chapter.

I agree with Gabbard and Westen (2003) that therapeutic action is no longer a question of interpretation vs. the relationship; instead it is a series of negotiations, clarifications, and emotional connections. I agree that therapeutic action cannot be defined in any singular way. However, fundamental to their view of therapeutic action, to the

BCPSG's view, and to my own, is the neuroscience-informed notion of changing neural pathways laid down in the brain. This is the basis for achieving affect regulation and is accomplished through a series of repetitive emotional events in treatment. These include recalling past affect-laden events repeatedly, but with each recall event, becoming better able to name, express, and manage the accompanying feelings. Again, I agree with Krystal (1988) that all "psychopathology" is affective in nature and requires greater awareness and affect regulation to achieve a therapeutic outcome.

Although we have produced numerous theories and clinical examples of how treatment works, I believe there has to be an overriding concept that we are missing. How else can we explain that regardless of theory—be it psychoanalytic, behavioral, or integrative—therapists behave more similarly than otherwise and produce similar results? (The exception being the impact of longer-term treatments.) This homogeneity contradicts our preferred beliefs of uniqueness and mystery as overriding factors in analytic treatment. And I say this with the knowledge that all treatment relationships are inherently unique. But is that uniqueness at the heart of therapeutic action, or is it something else? What activities can we engage in, what attitudes can we work toward displaying, what values can we hold, that are effective across patient populations?

First, and foremost, we must begin with a good match and therapist who has the general basic character structure outlined earlier. Formal training and personal treatment are also "required" in most cases, especially for a full analysis. These comments may seem superfluous and obvious, yet I have been surprised at how many psychodynamic therapists have not had their own treatment and/or who treat people they dislike from the start.

Second is the longstanding and popular view of providing a safe and empathic environment, marked by gentle curiosity and empathy. In my own treatment, I marveled at the sheer amount of time that analysis afforded me to explore my deepest thoughts and feelings. It was an experience like no other. Add in my analyst's empathic and intense attention, and I felt like I had entered another universe. So I often wonder to what extent this time and attention, in and of itself, has therapeutic value. To experience this over time is unique to those who pursue psychoanalysis. Therefore, I agree with those who emphasize empathic listening and an atmosphere of safety as essential prerequisites for change. Establishing safety and trust allows for both the revelation of shameful secrets and the ability to tolerate conflict.

Third, the observance of proper boundaries and patient education about the process are essential during this initial period of treatment and constitute a version of informed consent. I include in this a description of how and why focusing on emotion is important. Although we are loath to describe our technical approach, Barnicot et al. (2014) note the therapy research revealing that the more the patient knows what to expect, the better.

> Wampold and Budge (2012), in which they argue that patients' initial trust in the working relationship with their clinicians is hugely bolstered if clinicians provide a credible theory to explain the source of patients' problems and then prescribe the use of specific techniques to resolve them (p. 115).

You might argue that psychoanalysts do not possess "specific techniques," nor do they wish to. We certainly do not use manuals, nor will we ever be doing so. However, in the context of analysis, explaining things like free association, transference-countertransference, and the importance of experiencing emotion for the change process are all examples of what we are either already doing or could implement in an organized way. We could also recognize the value of patient education and agreed-upon treatment goals in a more formal way during analytic training.

Fourth, in the interests of determining what is and isn't therapeutic, I think we could identify types of interventions that work better than others. For example, the research has demonstrated what most of us would consider obvious: Hostile comments and criticism are not therapeutic. But I think we can do better than that. Supervisees ask me questions like, "I have a patient who doesn't like me to ask direct questions because it reminds of her interrogating mother. But how else can I clarify what she is saying, especially if I am not sure?"

Since specific interventions are beyond the scope of this chapter, suffice it to say that I provided her with more open-ended statements that have a softer tone. The whole area of expressing negative emotions, as I outlined earlier in this volume, is very controversial, but I have created guidelines (Maroda, 1991, 2010) that are general enough to work for anyone. Needless to say, these interventions fall squarely in the realm of conscious, verbal exchanges that are critical to the analytic process. I agree with Levin (2011) who, citing Lichtenberg, says,

> We are working in an era in which the pendulum in analytic theorizing on therapeutic action has swung from a focus on verbalization to a focus on implicit, often ineffable, nonverbal processes like relational interconnectedness, the container function, moments of meeting, disciplined spontaneous engagements, empathic immersion, the resolution of enactments, and dissociation, the repair of ruptures, and the role of the "the third" as variously theorized. Perhaps, Lichtenberg thought, not enough is being said these days about how the words and wording that we choose in speaking to our patients contribute to the therapeutic action of analytic process. (p. 1221)

I would add to this mix the value of renewed concentration on the use of metaphor, a once highly valued concept in psychoanalysis that has become controversial in recent years because it relies on the analyst's interpretation of the patient's experience.

Fifth is the complex set of behaviors involved in recognizing how analyst and patient are recreating their established ways of feeling and behaving with each other. The literature on transference-countertransference is too exhaustive to cover here. Much has been written about the transference and the countertransference, but too little about how these two forces seamlessly merge or collide. The concept of enactment is an attempt to understand the complex patterns of interaction between analyst and patient, but does so in a manner that focuses primarily on the unknown. How do we harness the power of these light and dark forces as they play out between us and our patients?

I have focused my own work on the role of the analyst in *completing the cycle of affective communication*, which I mentioned earlier. If one accepts that emotion is the currency of therapeutic action, then it is incumbent upon us to deal more directly with the emotion that flows through the analytic dyad. Doing so requires a high level of self-awareness in the analyst, requiring the aforementioned relinquishment of our claims on "goodness" in favor of authenticity. In a meta-analysis of treatment outcome, Diener et al. (2007) conclude, "Our results indicate that the more therapists facilitate the affective experience/expression of patients in psychodynamic therapy, the more patients exhibit positive changes" (p. 939). Although their research did not include any specific techniques for facilitating the patient's affect, nor what types of affective expression are most helpful, these results are congruent with my own theory of affective communication. And I continue to believe that our avoidance of conflict and negative emotions in the transference-countertransference represent a huge obstacle to mining many of the deep affective experiences our patients need to have with us.

I am consistently impressed with how often both my patients and myself are relieved by some exchange centered on observing each other's negative emotions or missteps. And the sooner I recognize and give over to their perceptions of my intentions or mood, the better. They know who we really are, just as we know who they are, but they feel compelled to protect us from the truth if we do not readily accept it from them. Therapist patients, in particular, are hypervigilant and overly protective of their analysts as they were with their parents. Admitting to missteps or insensitivities does not necessarily make us vulnerable in the moment. Our vulnerability is more likely to become evident to us and to our patients when we are unexpectedly hurt and/or angry in response to something the patient says. It is these clutch moments described so well by Chused (2003) that determine whether or not we can be authentic. The fact that the patient has pushed our buttons, whether intentionally or unintentionally, is not lost on them. The extent that we ignore or deny our vulnerability in those moments determines how safe patients can feel to express themselves going forward.

Equally, our willingness to express negative feelings to our patients provides essential feedback and relief for them. As in the examples I have provided throughout this volume, patients who provoke negative feelings over time with us are probably doing the same with others. Often, they openly admit this and ask us to be honest with them.

I believe the essence of therapeutic action resides in the constructive and deliberate truth-telling within the analytic relationship.

Factors that need to be recognized include the desire to influence, the desire to change each other, the range of feelings we experience with each other, and the inevitable periods of withdrawal that occur. In short, it is the gradual awakening of who we are in relation to each other that is therapeutic, with the ongoing prominent focus on the patient. Grieving losses, missed opportunities, failures, and the fact of his limitations are all therapeutic if done at the proper time. This includes the harsh realities of abuse and not experiencing love. As Bell (2016) says,

> For you to accept that you've suffered certain kinds of bad experiences that have had an inescapable effect upon you, that you will live with for the rest of our life, can have a curious form of freeing. That's what I am. That's what I'm like. I hope to develop. But I can't aim to develop to transcend my history, my cultural location, the way I've been genderised as an individual in a family, socially and culturally. (p. 9)

What Bell and others know is that relational freedom emanates from simply accepting what is. As D. B. Stern (2013) says, "Relational freedom makes the freedom to experience possible, and therefore underpins therapeutic action" (p. 234). Therapeutic action is not about changing who we are or what happened to us; it is about going through the painful process of recognizing, emoting, regulating, and accepting who we are.

Pattern recognition in the dyad

Ablon and Jones (2005) have done some fascinating preliminary research on the repetition of patterns across treatments. They identified what they called "interaction structures," which incorporate the repetitive patterns characteristic of each person, along with the reality of their attempts to mutually influence each other. The authors report that these patterns were stable over time, which fits with the ideas presented here. Any change was slow and was the result of repeated negotiations. Even though the reality of the uniqueness of any relationship cannot be denied, neither can the reality of our stable patterns of thinking, feeling, and behaving that we bring to every relationship.

Pattern recognition, which was the basis for the now unpopular practice of diagnosis, has its value. Although it can result in inappropriate and dehumanizing generalizations and biases, it is how we recognize the world around us. It is also how we predict what will happen next. And the value of this predictive potential is a neglected aspect of analytic treatment. Schlesinger (2003) made the case that we should be in the business of thoughtful interventions that involve predicting how the patient is likely to react, rather than relying on unconscious determinants.

Therefore, I think it would behoove us to focus more on our own recurrent patterns and look for their repetition in each treatment situation, as many others have said. I think we would also do well to pay attention to what patients identify as their own patterns and track those as well. Therapeutic action is highly dependent on self-awareness and the emotional exchanges that occur as our "interactive structures" collide in treatment. As trained mental health professionals, we are in a position to facilitate encounters that are unlikely to occur elsewhere. Thus, our value does not lie primarily in our good character, as valuable as that may be. Our ultimate value lies in our ability to know ourselves, know our patients, and possess the knowledge and experience to facilitate the understanding of what happens between us.

Conclusion

Therapeutic action has defied definition throughout the history of psychoanalysis. This void has been perpetuated by a number of factors, including the lack of formal research; the current preference for focusing on unconscious processes and the unknown; the analyst's need to see him/herself as the good parent who repairs the patient's early childhood deficits; and analysts' reluctance to disclose what they actually say and do in treatment.

Gabbard and Westen (2003) have argued for multiple theories of therapeutic action, accompanied by indicated clinical strategies, to address the diverse population of patients. I have agreed with the basic idea of customization of every treatment, but have presented an argument for both an overarching theory and general principles for engagement. In addition, I have critiqued the work of the Boston

Change Process Study Group, chiefly because of their current influence on theory and technique, noting areas of agreement and disagreement.

Identifying and analyzing longstanding patterns of feeling and acting, both in patients and analysts, is highlighted as an essential feature in therapeutic action. The analyst's role is thus shifted from being a better person than the patient's caregivers to being someone uniquely capable of acknowledging and navigating what emerges between them.

Notes

1 See Barsness (2018) for a complete review and discussion of the research on psychodynamic treatment and its effectiveness.
2 For a more comprehensive review of the literature on therapeutic action, I recommend Abend (2007); Diamond and Christian (2011); Gabbard and Westen (2003); Lichtenberg (2012); Rangell (1992); Smith (2007); and Stern (1996).

References

Ablon, S. J., & Jones, E. E. (2005). On analytic process. *Journal of the American Psychoanalytic Association, 53*, 541–568.

Abend, S. (2007). Therapeutic action in modern conflict theory. *Psychoanalytic Quarterly,* 1417–1442.

Ackerman, S. J., & Hilsenroth, M. J. (2003). A review of therapist characteristics and techniques positively impacting the therapeutic alliance. *Clinical Psychology Review, 23*, 1–33.

Allison, E., & Fonagy, P. (2016). When is truth relevant? *Psychoanalytic Quarterly, 85*, 275–303.

Aron, L. (2000). Self-reflexivity and the therapeutic action of psychoanalysis. *Psychoanalytic Psychology, 17*, 667–689.

Barnicot, K., Wampold, B., & Priebe, S. (2014). The effect of core clinician interpersonal behaviors on depression. *Journal of Affective Disorders, 167*, 112–117.

Barsness, R. (Ed.) (2018). *Core competencies of relational psychoanalysis: A guide to practice, study, and research.* London Routledge.

Bell, D. (2016). David Bell on "Is truth an illusion? Psychoanalysis and postmodernism." *PED/UCL Top Authors Project, 1*, 9.

Benjamin, J. (1997). Psychoanalysis as a vocation. *Psychoanalytic Dialogues, 7*, 781–802.

Black, M. (2003). Enactment: Analytic musings on energy, language, and personal growth. *Psychoanalytic Dialogues, 13*, 633–655.

Blagys, M. D., & Hilsenroth, M. J. (2000). Distinctive activities of short-term psychodynamic-interpersonal psychotherapy: A review of the comparative psychotherapy process literature. *Clinical Psychology: Science and Practice, 7*, 167–188.

Blass, R.B. (2003). On ethical issues at the foundation of the debate over the goals of psychoanalysis. *International Journal of Psychoanalysis, 84*, 929–943.

Blass, R. (2010). Affirming 'That's not psycho-analysis!' On the value of the politically incorrect act of attempting to define the limits of our field. *International Journal of Psycho-Analysis, 91*, 81–99.

Boston Change Process Study Group. (2007). The foundational level of psychodynamic meaning: Implicit process in relation to conflict, defense and the dynamic unconscious. *International Journal of Psychoanalysis, 88*, 843–860.

Boston Change Process Study Group. (2018a). Engagement and the emergence of a charged other. *Contemporary Psychoanalysis, 54*, 540–559.

Boston Change Process Study Group. (2018b). Moving through and being moved by: Embodiment in development and in the therapeutic relationship. *Contemporary Psychoanalysis, 54*, 299–321.

Chused, J. F. (2003). The role of enactments. *Psychoanalytic Dialogues, 13*: 677–687.

Cornelius, J. T. (2018). The case for psychoanalysis: Exploring the scientific evidence. In R. Barsness (Ed.), *Core competencies in relational psychoanalysis* (pp. 24–42). London: Routledge.

Crastnopol, M. (2019). The analyst's Achilles' heels: Owning and offsetting the clinical impact of our intrinsic flaws. *Contemporary Psychoanalysis, 55*, 399–427.

Diamond, M. J., & Christian, C. (Eds.) (2011) *Evolving perspectives on therapeutic action: The second century of psychoanalysis*. London: Karnac Books.

Diener, M. J., Hilsenroth, M. J., & Weinberger, J. (2007). Therapist affect focus and patient outcomes in psychodynamic psychotherapy: A metaanalysis. *American Journal of Psychiatry, 164*, 936–941. DOI:10.1176/ajp. 2007.164.6.936.

Ellman, S. J., & Moskowitz, M. (1998). *Enactment: Toward a new approach to the therapeutic relationship*. New York: Jason Aronson.

Ellman, S. J., & Moskowitz, M. (2008). A study of the Boston Change Process Study Group. *Psychoanalytic Dialogues, 18*, 812–837.

Feiner, A. H., & Levenson, E. A. (1968–69). The compassionate sacrifice: An explanation of a metaphor. *Psychoanalytic Review, 55*, 552–573.

Fonagy, P. (2003). Some complexities in the relationship of psychoanalytic theory to technique. *Psychoanalytic Quarterly, 72*, 13–47.

Frank, K. A., & Bernstein, K. (2012). Therapeutic action: An introduction and overview. *Psychoanalytic Perspectives, 9*, 1–19.

Friedman, L. (2008). Is there life after enactment? The idea of the patient's proper work. *Journal of the American Psychoanalytic Association, 56*, 431–453.

Gabbard, G. O., & Westen, D. (2003). Rethinking therapeutic action. *International Journal of Psychoanalysis, 84*, 823–841.

Hirsch, I. (1983). Analytic intimacy and the restoration of nurturance. *American Journal of Psychoanalysis, 43*, 325–343.

Hirsch, I. (2008). *Coasting in the countertransference: Conflicts of self-interest between analyst and patient.* New York: The Analytic Press.

Kantrowitz, J. (1993). The uniqueness of the patient-analyst pair: Approaches for elucidating the analyst's role. *International Journal of Psychoanalysis, 74*, 893–904.

Kantrowitz, J. (2002). The external observer and the lens of the patient-analyst match. *International Journal of Psychoanalysis, 83*, 339–350.

Kravis, N. (2013). The analyst's hatred of analysis. *Psychoanalytic Quarterly, 82*, 89–114.

Krystal, H. (1988). *Integration and self-healing: Affect, trauma, alexithymia.* Hillsdale, NJ: The Analytic Press.

Levin, C. B. (2011). The analyst's words and wording: Do they still matter? *Journal of the American Psychoanalytic Association, 59*, 1221–1237.

Lingiardi, V., Muzi, L., Tanzilli, A., & Nicola, C. (2018). Do therapists' subjective variables impact on psychodynamic psychotherapy outcomes? A systematic literature review. *Clinical Psychology & Psychotherapy, 25*, 85–101.

Lichtenberg, J. (2012). Therapeutic action" Old and new explanations of therapeutic leverage. *Psychoanalytic Inquiry, 32*, 50–59.

Loewald, H. (1960). On the therapeutic action of psycho-analysis. *International Journal of Psychoanalysis, 41*, 16–33.

Maroda, K. (1991). *The power of countertransference: Innovations in analytic technique.* Chichester, UK: Wiley.

Maroda, K. (1999). *Seduction, surrender and transformation: Emotional engagement in the analytic process.* Hillsdale, NJ: The Analytic Press.

Maroda, K. (2010). *Psychodynamic techniques: Working with emotion in the therapeutic relationship.* New York: Guilford.

Mitchell, S. A. (1997). *Influence and autonomy in psychoanalysis.* Hillsdale, NJ: The Analytic Press.

Mitchell, S. A. (1988). *Relational concepts in psychoanalysis: An integration.* Cambridge, MA: Harvard University Press.

Modell, A. H. (2008). Implicit or unconscious? Commentary on paper by the Boston Change Process Study Group. *Psychoanalytic Dialogues, 18,* 162–167.

Panksepp, J. (1994). Subjectivity may have evolved in the brain as a simple value-coding process that promotes learning of new behaviors. In P. Eckman & R. Davidson (Eds.). *The nature of emotion: Fundamental questions* (pp. 313–315). New York: Oxford University Press.

Rangell, L. (1992). The psychoanalytic theory of change. *The International Journal of Psychoanalysis, 73,* 415–428.

Safran, J. D. (2003). The relational turn, the therapeutic alliance and psychotherapy research: Strange bedfellows or postmodern marriage? *Contemporary Psychoanalysis, 39,* 449–475.

Schlesinger, H. J. (2003). *The texture of treatment: On the matter of psychoanalytic technique.* Hillsdale, NJ: The Analytic Press.

Schore, A. N. (1994). *Affect regulation and the origin of the self: The neurobiology of emotional development.* Hillsdale, NJ: Lawrence Erlbaum Associates.

Searles, H. (1973). Concerning therapeutic symbiosis. *Annual of Psychoanalysis, 1,* 247–262.

Shedler, J. (2010). The efficacy of psychodynamic psychotherapy. *American Psychologist, 65,* 98–109.

Smith, H. F. (2007). In search of a theory of therapeutic action. *Psychoanalytic Quarterly, 76S* (Supplement), 1735–1761.

Stern, D. B. (1996). The social construction of therapeutic action. *Psychoanalytic Inquiry, 16,* 265–293.

Stern, D. B. (2013). Relational freedom and therapeutic action. *Journal of the American Psychoanalytic Association, 61,* 227–255.

Stern, D. N. (1985). *The interpersonal world of the infant.* New York: Basic Books.

Stern, D. N., Sander, L. W., Nahum, J. P., Harrison, A. M., Lyons-Ruth, K., Morgan, A. C., Brunschweiler-Stern, N., & Tronick, E. Z. (1998). Non-interpretive mechanisms in psychoanalytic therapy: The "something more" than interpretation. *International Journal of Psychoanalysis, 79,* 903–921.

Strachey, J. (1934). The nature of therapeutic action in psychoanalysis. *International Journal of Psychoanalysis, 15,* 127–159.

Vivona, J. (2006). From developmental metaphor to developmental model: The shrinking role of language in the talking cure. *Journal of the American Psychoanalytic Association, 54*, 877–902.

Vivona, J. (2009). Leaping from brain to mind: A critique of mirror neuron explanations of countertransference. *Journal of the American Psychoanalytic Association, 57*, 525–550.

Vivona, J. (2019). The interpersonal words of the infant: Implications of current infant language research for psychoanalytic theories of infant development, language, and therapeutic action. *Psychoanalytic Quarterly, 88*, 685–725.

Wampold, B. E., & Budge, S. L. (2012). The 2011 Leona Tyler Award Address: The relationship—And its relationship to the common and specific factors of psychotherapy. *The Counseling Psychologist*, 40(4), 601–623.

Conclusion

As I ponder my concluding statements, I feel an ambivalence toward using the word "conclusion." The point of this book was to bring suppressed feelings and hidden thoughts to the surface. It was to encourage people to say what they really feel and think without guilt or shame. It was to provoke engagement and debate. It was to bring down the totem of perfection and embrace our ordinary, and extraordinary, humanity. It was to promote healthy debate and skepticism.

I have taken great issue with our tendency toward passivity and conflict avoidance. This book will have accomplished its mission if the reader comes, not necessarily to my conclusions, but to the opening up of their own new thoughts and recognition of desires. Conclusions are meant to be challenged. Nonetheless, we need them because they provide the essential framework for defining who we are, what we know, and what we stand for. The next generation of analysts and therapists, as I have repeatedly said, need a body of theory and practice so they can learn what to do, and what not to do. They will necessarily modify those theories and techniques as needed to assert their own voice, the voices of their patients, and the voices of their generation.

But they need to know where to start. They need to know what we actually think and do. They need to know what has proven to be helpful and what has not. They need a framework within which they can begin their journey. We do not need to protect them from our convictions. They are perfectly capable of coming up with their own ideas if we provide an environment that encourages taking a stand, being creative, and truly engaging in dialogue. The sanest voices will prevail if we create an atmosphere that encourages them to be heard.

Index

Note: Page numbers followed by 'n' indicate note section.

Abend, S. 91, 205n2
Ablon, S. J. 203
Ackerman, S. J. 172
Ahadi, S. A. 160
Akhtar, S. 40
Albein-Urios, N. 145, 148
Alford, C. F. 38
Allison, E. 192
ambivalence 8, 10, 11, 13, 16; toward
  technique 15–17
analyst(s)
  desire to influence 104–105
  early experiences 5, 6, 7, 9, 14, 15, 18,
  25, 26, 28, 29, 46, 47, 49, 50, 65, 73–74,
  93, 100–101, 114, 172, 180, 185
  false self 103–108
  fear of doing harm 5–6, 9–10, 18
  gender and narcissism 77–79
  as good object 20–22, 24
  gratification 33–37, 50–60, 64
  guilt 6–7, 11, 13, 14, 15, 18, 22, 29, 36,
  68, 70, 83, 100, 173
  motivations 18–19
  narcissistic injury 65
  narcissistic vulnerability 65
  needs 18; managing therapist's 33–38,
  50–51; narcissistic 64–67, 72, 75–77;
  selfobject 50, 52
  negative feelings (countertransference)
  100, 111–114
  managing within conflict 111–114, 125
  therapist's use of 129
  threat posed by 108–111
  passivity 13–15, 19
  persona 21

sacrifice 33; self-sacrificing 38–41
self-disclosure 120
shame 10, 13, 15, 18, 22–24, 34, 36, 52,
  58–59, 65, 66, 70, 73, 83, 173
transformation 53, 56
vulnerability 22–25, 64–66, 68–71
analytic desires 103
approach motives 42–43
Arizmendi, T. G. 149, 151
Aron, L. 28, 52, 56, 91, 101, 121,
  125, 186
Arriage, X. B. 41
asymmetry 105
Atlas, G. 125
Atwood, G. 26
avoidance motives 42

Bacal, H. 49, 52
Bargh, J. A. 127, 128
Barnicot, K. 188, 196, 200
Barrett, L. F. 146, 147
Barsness, R. 195, 204
Bass, A. 121
Batson, C. D. 149
Beebe, B. 107–108
Bell, D. 202
Bellak, L. 53
Bekkali, S. 145, 148
Bekkering, H. 149
Benjamin, J. 26, 195
Bergman, A. 95
Berlin, H. A. 127
Bernstein, K. 182
Bird, B. 112
Black, M. 137, 182

Blagys, M. D. 195
Blass, R.B 194
Blass, R. 142
Blau, P. M. 42
Boesky, D. 120
Bohleber, W. 119–120, 122
Bolding, J. 144
Bolognini, S. 163
Booth, L. 160
borderline personality disorder 14, 44
Boston Change Process Study Group
    125, 127, 146, 147, 148, 163, 190–194
Bowlby, J. 95
Brenner, C. 7, 51, 91
Bromberg, P. 26
Brothers, L. 150
Brunschweiler-Stern, N. 191
Budge, S. L. 199
Buechler, S. 22
Busch, F. 92, 119
Buysse, A. 159

Carmeli, Z. 142
Celenza, A. 7, 43, 100, 105–106
Christian, C. 89, 90–91, 204
Christov-Moore, L. 145
Chused, J. 64, 65, 76, 125–127,
    130–131, 202
Coen, S. 35, 73–74
conflict 89; and analyst's negative
    feelings 111–114; avoidance of 127
    brief history of 90–91; failure to
    address 101; modern conflict theory 91;
    in relational theory 91–95; use of 129
Cooper, A. 26
Cornelius, J. T. 195
countertransference 12, 21–24, 27, 89,
    91, 99, 110, 111–114, 124–125
Cox, C. L. 41
Craig, K. D. 159
Craighero, L. 142
Craik, F. I. 160
Crastnopol, M. 56, 174
Csibra, G. 142, 149

Damasio, A. R. 151
Davila, J. 15
Decety, J. 152, 153, 160
"developmental tilt" 94–97, 164
Diamond, M. J. 204
Diener, M. J. 195, 201
disengagement 130

Donaldson, P. H. 145, 148
Downey, G. et al 42
Drigotas, S. M. 41
Dunbar, N. E. 107

Eagle, M. 67, 147, 148, 159
Ellman, S. J. 192
emotional engagement 14–15
enactment 67, 89, 109–111; definition of
    119; pitfalls of 131; role of
    consciousness in 137
Enticott, P. G. 145, 148
empathy: beyond empathy 163–166;
    challenges to being empathic 161–163;
    definition and problematic uses in
    analytic theory and practice 151–154;
    extreme 96; limitations of 157–160;
    mirror neuron development in
    144–146; myths about 141
Engen, H. G. 160
Englis, B. G. 161
Erikson, E. H. 103

facial mimicry 148
Fairbairn, W. R. D. 95
Faithorn, P. 53
Farber, B. 50, 77
fear of doing harm 9, 110, 123, 129
Feiner, A. H. 179
Ferenczi, S. 51
Fine, R. 55
Finell, J. 64
Fink, G. R. 161
Fonagy, P. 17, 119, 120, 122, 192
Frank, K. A. 182
Friedman, L. 186
Frommer, M. S. 71

Gabbard, G. 34, 43, 54–55, 57, 92,
    113, 121
Gabbard, G. O. 166, 186–188, 196,
    198, 204
Gable, S. L. 42, 43
Gallese, V. 142, 143, 147, 148, 159
Gelso, C. J. 15–16
Gerson, M. J. 14
Ghent, M. 38–39
Gill, M. M. 67
Ginot, E. 128
Glaser, J. 128
Goldfried, M. 15
Goldfried, M. R. 100

Goldman, A. 143
"good enough mother" 18, 19–20, 22, 24, 89, 97, 129
Goubert, L. 159
gratification 33–37, 43, 50–60, 64
Greenberg, J. 74
Grossman, L. 16–17
Grossmark, R. 137
guilt 6–7, 11, 13, 14, 15, 18, 22, 29, 34, 68, 70, 83, 100, 173
Guntrip, H. 95

Han, S. 158
Harris, A. 15, 52, 26, 91
Harrison, A. M. 191
Haselager, P. 149
Hassein, R. R. 127–128
Hayes, C. 15–16, 111
Hayes, J. A. 15–16
Heifetz, L. 50, 77
Hein, G. 152
Hepworth, M. (see Target, M.)
Herbette, G. 159
Herron, W. G. 75, 78, 101
Hershey, K. L. 160
Hickock, G. 142–143, 148, 149
Hilsenroth, M. J. 172, 195
Hirsch, I. 24, 65, 67, 97, 151, 175
Holtz, P. 107
Hyde, C. 145, 148

IARPP 14, 173
Impett, E.A. 42–43
implicit communication 119
influence: analyst's desire to 104–106; mutual influence 101, 121; of women 27–29
Ivey, G. 123

Jacobs, D. 25
Jacobs, T. 6, 26, 120–121, 125–126
Jennings, L. 21
Jimeniz, J. P. 119, 120, 122
Jones, E. E. 203
Jones, R. A. 12, 49, 64, 75, 77, 78

Kantrowitz, J. L. 18, 175–176, 181
Kihlstrom, J. F. 128
Kilborne, B. 71
Killgore, W.D.S 153
Kim, H. 158
Kite, J.V 6, 25

Knox, J. 157
Kohut, H. 76, 103, 154
Kravis, N. 40, 68–69, 78, 194
Kriegman, D. K. 101–102, 107
Krystal, H. 193, 198
Kuchuck, S. 77

Lachmann, F. 107–108
Lamm, C. 149, 160
Langs, R. 82
Lanzetta, J. T. 161
LeDoux, J. 96
Lerner, M. J. 42
Levenson, E. 27, 122
Levenson, E. A. 179
Levin, C. B. 200
Levinas, E. 38
Levenkron, H. 123
Lichtenberg, J.
Lingiardi, V. 197
Little, M. 21, 72
Livingston, M. 69
Loewald, H. 178, 182–183
Luchner, A. F. 12, 49, 64, 75, 77, 78
Lyons-Ruth, K. 191

Mahler, M. 95
Majdandzic, J. 149, 160
Manfredi Turillazzi, S. 164
Mark, D. 21
Markowitsch, H. J. 161
Maroda, K. 5, 9, 17, 26, 48, 51, 120, 129, 198, 200
match (therapeutic) 18, 171–175
McGilchrist, I. 145, 149
McLaughlin, J. 57, 113
McWilliams, N. 26
Mendolsohn, E. 21
Michalski, K. J. 153
Migone, P. 147, 148, 159
Miller, A. 12
Mills, J. 20, 29, 113–114
mirror neurons: adaption by psychoanalysis 146–150; controversy and history 142–144; relationship to empathy 144–146
Mirsalimi, H. 12, 49, 64, 75, 77, 78
Mitchell, S. A. 29, 52–53, 83, 91–97, 99, 103, 108–109, 114, 164, 179, 187
Modell, A. 111, 192
Morgan, A. C. 191
Mose, C. J. 12, 49, 64, 75, 77, 78

Moses, I. 164, 166
Moskowitz, M. 192
motivations 18–19
Muran, J. C. 22, 100, 111, 113, 189
mutuality 15–16, 51, 58; and influence
    101; mutual denial 106
Muzi, L. 197

Nahum, J. P. 191
narcissism 64–67, 72; gender and
    narcissism 77–79; healthy
    narcissism 75–77
needs 33–38, 50–51, 64
Nelson, D. L. B. 111
Nicola, C. 197
"not-knowing" 19–20, 194–195
Nunberg, H. 105

Ochsner, K. 145
Olinick, S. L. 6
Orange, D. 13, 38–40
Ormont, L. R. 113, 124

Panksepp, J. 192
passivity 13–15
pattern recognition 203
Peplau, L. A. 42, 43
persona 19, 21
personal information 123
personal distress 157, 158
Piefke, M. 161
Pine, F. 95
Pinksy, E. 24, 27, 41, 73
power 105–107
Priebe, S. 188, 196, 200
Prodgers, A. 11
projective identification 120–121
Psychoanalytic Dialogues 29
Pulver, S. 65, 142

Rangell, L. 183
Renik, O. 122, 131
Richards, A. 131
Righetti, F. 42
Rimé, B. 159
Rizzolatti, G. 142, 148, 151
Rosenblatt, P. 36
Rothbart, M. K. 160
Rusbult, C. E. 41

sacrifice 33; in close relationships 41–47;
    motivation for 41–43

Safran, J. 22, 111, 113, 189
Sandler, J. 137
Sander, L. W. 191
Scarfone, D. 119, 120, 122
Schlesinger, H. J. 203
Schore, A. N. 95
Schulte-Ruther, M. 161
Searles, H. F. 6, 9, 12, 24, 51, 112, 179
self-disclosure 119; definition of
    122–124, 127–128; uses of 129,
    136–137
self-object needs 49, 52
Seligson, A. G. 64
Shaker, A. 113
shame 10, 13, 15, 18, 22–24, 34, 36, 52,
    58–59, 65, 66, 70, 73, 83, 173
Shapiro, Y. 34
Shedler, J. 172
Shulman, M. 36
Singer, T. 152, 160
Sinigaglia, C. 148, 151
Skovholt, T. 21
Slavin, M. O. 101–102, 107
Slochower, J. 22, 103
Smith, H. F. 188
Solms, M. 112
Stern, D. B. 95, 164, 181, 203
Stern, D. N. 151, 191
Stolorow, R. 26
Steinberg, B. 26
Storr, A. 11
Strachey, J. 182
surrender 38
Sussman, M. 5–6, 34, 51, 64, 76
Szasz, T. 53–54

Tanzilli, A. 197
Target, M. 44–47
technique 15–17
theory as personal 25, 171
theory of mind 143, 146
therapeutic action 171–174, 178–179;
    contemporary issues in 186–190;
    history of 181–183; and "not
    knowing" 194–195; and pattern
    recognition 203; questioning the focus
    on the analyst 183–186; in relation to
    Boston Change Process Study Group
    190–194; "truth telling" 202
Thomson, P. 49, 52
transference-countertransference 21
transformation 53, 56

transition from classical to relational analysis 26–29
trauma patients 96
Tronick, E. Z. 21, 191

Uithol, S. 149
Uleman, J. S. 127, 128
unconscious 5–6, 13, 21, 46, 54, 60, 64, 91, 109–110, 119–121, 125, 127–128; to unconscious communication 146–147, 149–150

Van Lange, P. A. M. 41
van Rooij, I. 149
Varma, A. 40
Varvin, S. 119, 120, 122
Vivona, J. 142, 146–149, 157, 161, 192–193
vulnerability 21–23, 64–66, 68–71

Wachtel, P. 14 95, 122

Wampold, B. 188, 196, 200
Wampold, B. E. 200
Welt, S. R. 75, 78, 101
Westen, D. 166
Westen, D. 166, 186–188, 196, 198, 204
Wink, P. 76
Winnicott, D.W. 20–21, 93–97
Wilson, M. 50, 64, 75, 76, 103
Witcher, B. S. 41
Wolf, E. 52, 76
Wolf, A. W. 100
writing about patients 56–57

Youssef, G. J. 145, 148
Yurgelun-Todd, D. A. 153

Zaki, J. 145
Zelazo, P. D. 160
Zysman, S. 119, 120, 122

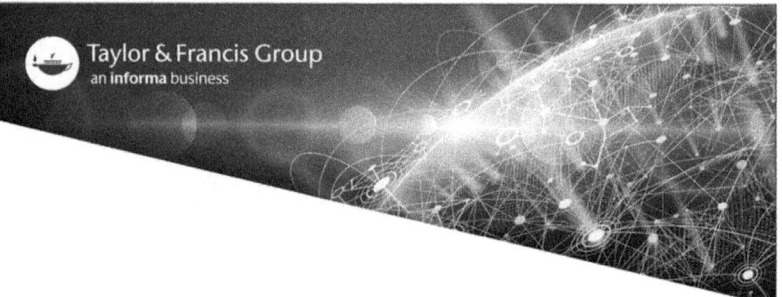
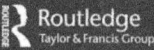
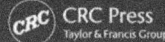

For Product Safety Concerns and Information please contact our EU
representative GPSR@taylorandfrancis.com
Taylor & Francis Verlag GmbH, Kaufingerstraße 24, 80331 München, Germany

www.ingramcontent.com/pod-product-compliance
Ingram Content Group UK Ltd.
Pitfield, Milton Keynes, MK11 3LW, UK
UKHW022259051225
465792UK00007B/110